MRCS Practice Papers
Part A: Paper 2
EMQs

Second edition

PasTest

Dedicated to your success

MRCS Practice Papers
Part A: Paper 2
EMQs

Second edition

Kim Lammin
BSc, MB ChB, MRCS
Specialist Registrar,
Trauma and Orthopaedics,
Royal Lancaster Infirmary
Lancaster

Jo Warner
MBChB
ST2 General Surgery
Royal Preston Hospital
North West Deanery

PasTest
Dedicated to your success

© 2009 PASTEST LTD

Egerton Court
Parkgate Estate
Knutsford
Cheshire
WA16 8DX

Telephone: 01565 752000

A percentage of questions were previously published in Intercollegiate MRCS: EMQ Practice Papers
First published 2006, Second edition 2009, Reprinted 2010

ISBN: 1 905635 621
ISBN: 978 1 905635 627

A catalogue record for this book is available from the British Library.

The information contained within this book was obtained by the authors from reliable sources. However, while every effort has been made to ensure its accuracy, no responsibility for loss, damage or injury occasioned to any person acting or refraining from action as a result of information contained herein can be accepted by the publishers or authors.

PasTest Revision Books and Intensive Courses

PasTest has been established in the field of postgraduate medical education since 1972, providing revision books and intensive study courses for doctors preparing for their professional examinations.

Books and courses are available for the following specialties:

MRCGP, MRCP Parts 1 and 2, MRCPCH Parts 1 and 2, MRCS, MRCOG, DRCOG, DCH, FRCA, PLAB Parts 1 and 2, Dental Students and Dentists.

For further details contact:

PasTest, Freepost, Knutsford, Cheshire WA16 7BR

Tel: 01565 752000   **Fax: 01565 650264**

www.pastest.co.uk   **enquiries@pastest.co.uk**

Text prepared by Carnegie Book Production, Lancaster

Printed and bound in the UK by CPI Antony Rowe

Contents

Foreword

This book is aimed at MRCS candidates and contains three complete practice papers.

The book has been written by people who recently sat the examination, and has been updated to reflect current question trends, with the aim of providing papers similar to those in the actual examination. Each paper covers the same variety of topics as laid out in the intercollegiate MRCS syllabus and the questions are of varying degrees of difficulty, in order to make the papers as similar to the exam as possible. Several topics are covered in more than one paper, reflecting the fact that these are frequently asked about.

The questions consist of a topic followed by a list of options and then the questions that are linked to that stem. Each answer can be used once, not at all or more than once.

The book aims to provide candidates with valuable practice at extended matching questions in advance of the exam, and to aid candidates in identifying areas of weakness for further study. It is designed to be used in conjunction with the recommended MRCS textbooks, and does not cover every topic.

We hope you will find this book useful.

Good Luck!

Kim and Jo

Examination technique

This is a brief guide which we hope you will find helpful for the EMQ paper of the MRCS.

Most of the points mentioned below are fairly obvious, but during the stress of the exam it is easy to forget some of them.

Revision

- Start revising early – you never have as much time as you think you do.
- Try to revise with someone else sitting the same exam.
- Do plenty of practice questions so that you are familiar with the format.

In the exam itself

- Read the instructions carefully.
- Allow enough time to complete the paper.
- If you are initially writing the answers on the questions sheet, make sure you allow time to transfer them to the answer sheet.
- Always turn over the last page – you wouldn't be the first person to miss the last few questions.
- Read the questions thoroughly.
- If the question seems too simple, it probably *is* that straightforward; there should not be any trick questions in the exam.

Good luck.

Abbreviations

A&E	Accident and Emergency
AAA	abdominal aortic aneurysm
ABPI	ankle–brachial pressure index
ACL	anterior cruciate ligament
ACTH	adrenocorticotropic hormone
AIN	anal intra-epithelial neoplasia
AP	anteroposterior
ASA	American Society of Anesthesiologists
ASB	assisted spontaneous breathing
BCG	bacille Calmette–Guérin
BIPAP	biphasic positive airway pressure
BMI	body mass index
BPH	benign prostatic hyperplasia
CEA	carcinoembryonic antigen
CIS	carcinoma in situ
CMV	continuous mandatory ventilation
CPAP	continuous positive airway pressure
CRP	C-reactive protein
CT	computed tomography
CVP	central venous pressure
DDH	developmental dysplasia of the hip
DRE	digital rectal examination
ECG	electrocardiogram
ESR	erythrocyte sedimentation rate
ESWL	extracorporeal shock-wave lithotripsy
FBC	full blood count
GCS	Glasgow Coma Scale

GGT   γ-glutamyl transferase
GTN   glyceryl trinitrate
hCG   human chorionic gonadotropin
HIV   human immunodeficiency virus
ICU   Intensive Care Unit
IVU   intravenous urogram
KUB   kidney-ureter-bladder (X-ray)
MEN   multiple endocrine neoplasia
MSU   mid-stream urine
NPV   negative predictive value
NSAID   non-steroidal anti-inflammatory drug
PCNL   percutaneous nephrolithotomy
PDS   polydioxanone suture
PEG   percutaneous endoscopic gastrostomy
PPV   positive predictive value
PSA   prostate-specific antigen
PTH   parathyroid hormone
RIF   right iliac fossa
RTA   road traffic accident
RUQ   right upper quadrant
SIMV   synchronous intermittent mandatory ventilation
SLE   systemic lupus erythematosus
SUFE   slipped upper femoral epiphysis
TPN   total parenteral nutrition
TURBT   transurethral resection of bladder tumour
TURP   transurethral resection of prostate
TWOC   trial without catheter
U&E   urea and electrolytes
UTI   urinary tract infection
VMA   vanillylmandelic acid
WCC   white cell count

QUESTIONS

QUESTIONS
PRACTICE PAPER 1

THEME: DIATHERMY

A Monopolar diathermy

B Bipolar diathermy

C Cutting

D Coagulation

E Blend

For each of the following scenarios, choose the most appropriate option from the list above. Each option may be used once, more than once or not at all.

1 Requires a patient plate electrode to be applied.

2 This is safer to use in patients with pacemakers.

3 Uses pulsed, short, high-frequency bursts.

4 Safe for use on digits.

5 Can be used for buzzing (touching other instruments to pass current through them).

THEME: EXTENSOR COMPARTMENTS OF THE WRIST

A I

B II

C III

D IV

E V

F VI

For each of the following statements, choose the most appropriate compartment from the list above. Each option may be used once, more than once or not at all.

O   6   Extensor carpi radialis brevis is in this compartment.

O   7   This compartment lies radial to Lister's tubercle at the wrist.

O   8   Extensor digiti minimi is in this compartment.

THEME: SEPSIS

A Bacteraemia

B Systemic inflammatory response syndrome (to sepsis) (SIRS)

C Sepsis

D Severe sepsis

E Septic shock

For each of the following clinical scenarios, choose the most appropriate diagnosis from the list above. Each option may be used once, more than once or not at all.

○ 9 A 30-year-old man presents with severe right loin pain, radiating to the groin. A mid-stream urine (MSU) shows blood, protein and nitrites. A KUB study reveals a calculus. His temperature is 39.1 °C, pulse 127/min, respiratory rate (RR) 38 breaths/min and BP 81/43 mmHg despite 3 litres of intravenous fluids, and his white cell count (WCC) is 21×10^9/l.

○ 10 A 79-year-old woman 1 week post-op has a pyrexia of 38.4 °C, pulse 104/min, BP 144/90 mmHg and WCC 14×10^9/l. Chest X-ray (CXR) shows a left lower lobe pneumonia.

○ 11 A 30-year-old male post-op patient had blood cultures taken 48 hours ago which are positive. He is currently apyrexial, pulse 64/min, RR 12 breaths/min, BP 123/82 mmHg, with a normal WCC.

○ 12 A 27-year-old female post-op patient has a temperature of 38.7 °C, pulse 86/min, RR 24 breaths/min, BP 127/74 mmHg and WCC 16×10^9/l. Her CXR is clear, an MSU negative and the wound is fine.

THEME: FACIAL NERVE PALSIES

A   Multiple sclerosis

B   Acoustic neuroma

C   Sarcoidosis

D   Choleasteatoma

E   Parotid tumour

F   Surgery

G   Temporal bone fracture

H   Ramsay Hunt syndrome

I   Chronic suppurative otitis media

J   Cerebrovascular accident (CVA)

K   Bell's palsy

For each of the following scenarios, choose the most appropriate option from the list above. Each option may be used once, more than once or not at all.

13   An 18-year-old man presents to A&E with a head injury. He has a facial nerve palsy, Battle's sign and haemotympanum.

14   A 30-year-old woman presents with a sudden-onset facial nerve palsy sparing the forehead. She has a past medical history of optic neuritis.

15   An 80-year-old man presents with a facial nerve palsy, preceded by severe pain in the distribution of the facial nerve. He reports vertigo and hearing loss. Papules are seen on the tongue.

16   A 50-year-old man presents with a facial nerve palsy. He has had an intermittent discharge from his right ear for 2 months. He has posterosuperior retraction of the tympanic membrane.

17   A 55-year-old woman presents with a facial nerve palsy, sensorineural hearing loss, tinnitus and vertigo.

18   A 23-year-old man presents with a facial nerve palsy and a 3-month history of conductive hearing loss. The tympanic membrane is dull in the left ear.

THEME: ANAESTHETIC AGENTS

A Thiopentone sodium

B Propofol

C Etomidate

D Suxamethonium

E Atracurium

F Vercuronium

G Halothane

H Enflurane

I Isoflurane

J Sevoflurane

K Nitrous oxide

For each of the following statements, choose the most appropriate agent from the list above. Each option may be used once, more than once or not at all.

19 Can cause a 'coronary steal' syndrome.

20 The most rapidly acting depolarising muscle relaxant.

21 The only inhalational anaesthetic not known to cause malignant hyperpyrexia.

22 The induction agent with a slight anti-emetic effect, which is the agent of choice with laryngeal masks.

THEME: FLEXOR TENDON INJURIES

A   Zone 1

B   Zone 2

C   Zone 3

D   Zone 4

E   Zone 5

For each of the following injuries, choose the most appropriate zone from the list above. Each option may be used once, more than once or not at all.

O   23   Laceration across both hypothenar and thenar eminences.

O   24   Most difficult to repair, often yielding poor functional outcome.

O   25   Laceration across the metacarpophalangeal (MCP) joints.

THEME: DAY-CASE SURGERY

A   Suitable for day-case surgery

B   Unsuitable for day-case surgery

For each of the following patients, choose the most appropriate option from the list above. Each option may be used once, more than once or not at all.

O   26   A 40-year-old woman listed for varicose vein stripping, with no significant past medical history. Weight 90 kg, height 155 cm. Her husband can look after her post-op and she lives 10 minutes from the hospital.

O   27   A 64-year-old with well-controlled asthma listed for rigid cystoscopy. Weight 74 kg, height 173 cm. He lives with his wife approximately 10 minutes form the hospital.

O   28   A 50-year-old man with angina requiring frequent GTN spray, listed for a knee arthroscopy. Weight 70 kg, height 180 cm. He lives with his wife approximately 5 minutes from the hospital.

THEME: URINARY SYSTEM TRAUMA

A Class I

B Class II

C Class III

D Class IV

E Class V

For each of the following scenarios, choose the most appropriate trauma class from the list above. Each option may be used once, more than once or not at all.

○ 29 An 18-year-old football player who sustained a kick to the loin during a game subsequently develops microscopic haematuria.

○ 30 A 30-year-old man who has been stabbed in the right loin with a kitchen knife arrives in A&E with a pulse of 112/min, BP 120/100 mmHg. He has frank haematuria. IVU reveals urinary extravasation.

○ 31 Following a hysterectomy a patient has macroscopic haematuria, ileus, pain and a low-grade fever. IVU reveals leakage from the left ureter. A 75% laceration with no devascularisation is found.

THEME: BURNS

A 10 800 ml

B 5400 ml

C 8640 ml

D 4320 ml .

E 17 280 ml

F 14 400 ml

For each of the following scenarios, choose the correct volume of fluid replacement required from the list above. Each option may be used once, more than once or not at all.

○ 32 A man weighing 80 kg is admitted as an emergency after being rescued from a house fire. He has red, painful, blistered burns to his right arm, chest and abdomen. How much fluid does he require over the first 24 hours following his injury?

○ 33 A 60-kg woman is admitted to A&E with extensive burns. Her left arm and leg have dry, white, painless burns, and her anterior torso has erythematous painful burns with blistering. How much fluid does she require over the first 8 hours after her injury?

○ 34 A 120-kg chef is involved in a fire at work. He has sustained red, painful, blistered burns to both his arms, and has erythematous areas to his chest that haven't blistered. How much fluid does he require for resuscitation over the first 8 hours after this injury?

○ 35 An 60-kg woman is involved in a house fire after falling asleep with a lit cigarette. She sustains full-thickness burns to both arms and legs, and partial-thickness burns to the front of her torso. How much fluid should she be given in the first 24 hours after this injury?

THEME: ANTI-EMETICS

A Cyclizine

B Metoclopromide

C Ondansetron

D Levomepromazine

E Haloperidol

For each of the following, choose the most appropriate anti-emetic from the list above. Each option may be used once, more than once or not at all.

○ 36 A selective 5-hydroxytryptamine antagonist, useful for preventing vomiting caused by cytotoxic drugs.

○ 37 A dopamine-receptor antagonist that acts in the chemoreceptor trigger zone (CTZ).

○ 38 An H1-receptor antagonist, most effective if given before the onset of nausea and vomiting.

○ 39 A non-phenothiazine antipsychotic used to combat vomiting caused by emetogenic anti-cancer drugs.

THEME: SURGICAL INCISIONS

A Lanz

B Kocher's

C McEvedy's

D Inguinal

E Lockwood's

F Gridiron

G Collar

For each of the following operations, choose the most appropriate incision from the list above. Each option may be used once, more than once or not at all.

○ 40   A 63-year-old lady presents with a lump in her right groin, lateral and inferior to the pubic tubercle. It is tender to palpation and irreducible, with erythema to the overlying skin. Which incision would you make for her emergency procedure?

○ 41   A 17-year-old girl presents with a 2-day history of right iliac fossa pain. She has a temperature 37.8 °C and has vomited twice. Her blood tests reveal: CRP 142 mg/l, WCC 14.6 × 10⁹/l. She requires an emergency operation. Which incision would you use?

○ 42   A 52-year-old man undergoes a laparoscopic cholecystectomy. During dissection around Calot's triangle, unusual anatomy is discovered and it is no longer safe to proceed laparoscopically and the procedure is converted to an open one. Which incision would you make?

○ 43   A 45-year-old lady with Graves' disease presents with a large goitre and wants to have her condition corrected as she is hoping to get pregnant within the next couple of years. Which incision would you make for her elective procedure?

THEME: ANATOMICAL RELATIONS

A Artery

B Nerve

C Vein

For each of the following, choose the most appropriate structure from the list of options above. Each option may be used once, more than once or not at all.

O   44   In the popliteal fossa, which structure lies the deepest?

O   45   In the cubital fossa, what is the most medial structure?

O   46   At the hilum of the kidney, what is the most anterior structure?

O   47   Of the femoral structures immediately inferior to the inguinal ligament, which structure lies most lateral?

THEME: URINARY TRACT INFECTIONS

A *Chlamydia*

B *Escherichia coli*

C *Klebsiella*

D *Mycobacterium tuberculosis*

E *Proteus* spp.

F *Schistosoma haematobium*

G *Streptococcus pneumoniae*

For each of the following scenarios, choose the most likely pathogen from the list above. Each option may be used once, more than once or not at all.

○ 48 A 26-year-old woman presents with ureteric colic. A KUB study reveals a staghorn calculus in the right kidney.

○ 49 A 32-year-old HIV-positive woman attends clinic with symptoms of recurrent UTIs. Multiple mid-stream urine specimens have been sent by her general practitioner and have only revealed sterile pyuria.

○ 50 A 35-year-old businessman presents with a first episode of frank haematuria. He has just returned from a business trip to Egypt.

THEME: DYSPHAGIA

A Achalasia

B Barrett's oesophagus

C Chagas' disease

D Diffuse oesophageal spasm

E Gastro-oesophageal reflux disease

F Oesophageal carcinoma

G Pharyngeal pouch

H Scleroderma

For each of the following scenarios, choose the most likely diagnosis from the list above. Each option may be used once, more than once or not at all.

51   A 72-year-old heavy smoker presents with dysphagia, retrosternal discomfort and new-onset hoarseness of voice.

52   A 43-year-old man presents with a recurrent sore throat and halitosis and complains of regurgitating undigested food.

53   A 45-year-old woman presents with dysphagia. Barium swallow shows a 'bird's beak' appearance of the lower oesophagus.

THEME: INCONTINENCE

A Bladder instability

B Bladder outlet obstruction

C Genuine stress incontinence

D Neurogenic incontinence

E Psychogenic incontinence

F Small bladder capacity

For each of the following scenarios, choose the most likely diagnosis from the list above. Each option may be used once, more than once or not at all.

54 A 78-year-old man presents with urinary leakage. This occurs on coughing or sneezing. On further questioning, he admits to decreasing urinary flow and increased frequency of micturition, with small volumes passed. In addition he reports symptoms of incomplete emptying.

55 A 43-year-old woman with known multiple sclerosis presents to clinic with urinary incontinence. She has had two children. She passes water every hour, but often does not have the urge to void. She currently wears 8–10 incontinence pads per day.

56 A 21-year-old woman presents with recurrent urinary tract infection. She passes urine every hour, but sometimes has such urgency that she cannot reach the toilet in time to prevent leakage. Flexible cystoscopy reveals interstitial cystitis.

57 A 38-year-old woman presents with urinary incontinence. This occurs on exercising, coughing or sneezing. She has had four children, all vaginal deliveries.

58 A 36-year-old man presents with occasional urinary incontinence. He gives a history of gonorrhoea, which was successfully treated 1 year ago. He has a reduced urinary flow rate, and a post-micturition bladder scan reveals a volume of 560 ml.

THEME: PRE-OPERATIVE INVESTIGATIONS

A Electrocardiogram (ECG)

B ECG + full bood count (FBC)

C ECG + FBC + urea and electrolytes (U&E)

D ECG + FBC + U&E + chest X-ray

E ECG + FBC + U&E + chest X-ray + lung function tests

F ECG + U&E

G No investigation required

For each of the following scenarios, choose the most appropriate minimum acceptable pre-operative investigations needed from the list above. Each option may be used once, more than once or not at all.

○ 59 A 55-year-old man presents with a distal radius fracture requiring open reduction and internal fixation. He is otherwise fit and well and is not taking any medication. His body mass index (BMI) is 26 kg/m^2 and he is a non-smoker.

○ 60 A 31-year-old man attends the pre-admission clinic. He is to undergo elective inguinal hernia repair. He has had a recent chest infection but is otherwise fit and well. He is not taking any medication.

○ 61 A 61-year-old man is to undergo total hip replacement. He is otherwise healthy and is a non-smoker.

○ 62 A 66-year-old man is admitted for elective repair of a left inguinal hernia. His past medical history includes hypercholesterolaemia and hypertension. He is on diuretics.

○ 63 A 53-year-old woman is admitted for elective laparoscopy. Her past medical history is of asthma.

○ 64 A 49-year-old woman with hypertension, a non-smoker, is admitted for elective varicose vein surgery.

THEME: TREATMENT OF ULCERS

A Compression bandaging

B Debridement

C Excision

D Revascularisation

E Total contact casting

For each of the following scenarios, choose the most appropriate treatment option from the list above. Each option may be used once, more than once or not at all.

65 A 38-year-old type 1 diabetic patient presents with a deep ulcer over the head of the first metatarsal. It is painless and on further examination he has decreased sensation in the whole of the foot.

66 A 65-year-old presents with a large circumferential ulcer just above the medial malleolus. She has marked lipodermatosclerosis around the ulcer. Her ankle–brachial pressure index (ABPI) is 0.56.

67 A 71-year-old presents with a large circumferential ulcer over the shin. There is a smaller ulcer over the medial malleolus. The leg has an inverted champagne bottle appearance. A duplex scan shows patent deep veins and good flow in the posterior tibial and dorsalis pedis arteries.

68 A 69-year-old smoker has had a long-standing ulcer on the medial aspect of his right leg. It measures 4 cm in diameter. Recently it has become increasingly friable. The edges are thickened and raised and on further examination he has palpable right inguinal lymph nodes.

69 A 71-year-old heavy smoker attends clinic with a painful, deep, punched-out ulcer on the dorsum of his right foot. On inspection he has some hair loss on the right shin compared with the left, and the right leg is cool to touch.

THEME: SURGICALLY IMPORTANT ORGANISMS

A *Acinetobacter*

B *Bacteroides fragilis*

C *Escherichia coli*

D Fusobacteria

E *Klebsiella* spp.

F *Pseudomonas aeruginosa*

G *Staphylococcus aureus*

H *Staphylococcus epidermidis*

For each of the following scenarios, choose the most likely organism from the list above. Each option may be used once, more than once or not at all.

○ 70 A 34-year-old man has been on the intensive care unit (ICU) for 4 weeks. He has had multiple infections and is being treated with different antibiotics. He begins to show signs of multi-system infection, including meningitis.

○ 71 A 64-year-old man had a knee replacement 2 months ago. He complains of persistent pain, and X-rays appear to show some loosening of the prosthesis. An aspiration of the joint yields a coagulase-negative staphylococcus.

○ 72 A 34-year-old develops severe sepsis 5 days after pan-proctocolectomy for severe ulcerative colitis. Blood cultures reveal an anaerobe which is penicillin-resistant.

○ 73 A 19-year-old man attends with a large tonsillar abscess. Bacteriological examination reveals a Gram-negative rod-shaped organism.

○ 74 A 74-year-old with a chronic venous leg ulcer develops an infection within the ulcer. Bacteriological examination reveals a Gram-negative bacillus.

THEME: CORD LESIONS

A Anterior cord syndrome

B Brown–Séquard syndrome

C Cauda equina

D Central cord syndrome

E Posterior cord syndrome

For each of the following scenarios, choose the most likely diagnosis from the list above. Each option may be used once, more than once or not at all.

75 A 34-year-old man suffers a knife injury to the back. He is unable to move his left lower limb, and is complaining of severe pain from a further stab injury to the left leg. He is insensate to temperature on the right leg.

76 A 37-year-old woman falls from a horse. She describes a hyperextension-type injury and is ataxic.

77 A 64-year-old man falls down a flight of stairs. He is unable to move his right lower leg and cannot feel sharp instruments on the right leg. He still is able to feel coarse touch. X-rays reveal a compression fracture of T12.

78 A 76-year-old man walks into the A&E department. He complains of bilateral upper limb weakness after a fall in the morning. Initial cervical spine X-rays show marked degenerative changes.

THEME: BENIGN ANO-RECTAL CONDITIONS

A Delorme's procedure

B Diltiazem ointment

C Surgical haemorrhoidectomy

D Conservative treatment

E Lidocaine gel

F Rubber-band ligation

G Seton drainage

H Steroid enema

For each of the following scenarios, choose the most appropriate treatment from the list above. Each option may be used once, more than once or not at all.

○ 79 A 79-year-old woman presents with a prolapsed rectum.

○ 80 A 29-year-old man presents with pain on defecation and some fresh bleeding. He gives a history of recurrent constipation. There is a skin tag present at the 12-o'clock position. Digital rectal examination is normal but painful, and proctoscopy cannot be performed due to patient discomfort.

○ 81 A 27-year-old woman presents to clinic 2 months after childbirth. She complains of faeces streaked with fresh blood.

○ 82 A 43-year-old man complains of itching around the anus. He also admits to anal pain and occasional purulent discharge from the anus. Proctoscopy reveals a fistula beginning at the dentate line, travelling an intersphincteric route.

THEME: PAIN IN THE RIGHT UPPER QUADRANT

A Acute pancreatitis

B Ascending cholangitis

C Biliary colic

D Cholecystitis

E Chronic pancreatitis

F Empyema

G Lower lobe pneumonia

H Perforated peptic ulcer

I Pulmonary embolism

J Subphrenic abscess

For each of the following scenarios, choose the most appropriate option from the list above. Each option may be used once, more than once or not at all.

○ 83 A 40-year-old presents with intermittent right upper quadrant (RUQ) pain radiating to the back. It is associated with nausea and vomiting. The patient is not obviously jaundiced, but has dark urine. The patient is apyrexial.

○ 84 A 43-year-old man presents with severe RUQ pain radiating to the back. He is visibly jaundiced and complains of chills and rigors. There are calculi in the gallbladder on ultrasound, but none in the common bile duct.

○ 85 A 60-year-old woman with known diverticular disease, who was previously admitted 1 month ago, presents with nausea, weight loss, anaemia, rigors and a raised WCC.

○ 86 A 30-year-old man presents with severe RUQ pain radiating to the back, associated with vomiting. His amylase is 1520 Somogyi U/dl.

87 A 25-year-old man presents with RUQ pain and pyrexia, but no rigors. He has a raised WCC, normal findings on liver function tests and normal amylase. Ultrasound scan is normal.

THEME: VENTILATORS

A Assisted spontaneous breathing (ASB)

B Biphasic positive airway pressure (BIPAP)

C Continuous mandatory ventilation (CMV)

D Continuous positive airways pressure (CPAP)

E High-frequency jet ventilation

F Positive end-expiratory pressure

G Synchronous intermittent mandatory ventilation (SIMV)

For each of the following statements, choose the most appropriate form of ventilation from the list above. Each option may be used once, more than once or not at all.

88 The form of ventilation used to assist a patient's inspiratory effort. It is used to effectively 'top-up' a patient's own volume of inspired air.

89 The most frequently used form of ventilation in theatre. It can be set to pressure- or volume-controlled mode.

90 The form of ventilation used in spontaneously breathing patients to splint the alveoli and improve respiratory mechanics.

91 The form of ventilation used to help wean patients from ventilators. Breaths are synchronised with the patient's respiratory efforts.

THEME: MANAGEMENT OF CHEST TRAUMA

A   Application of three-sided occlusive dressing

B   Cardiopulmonary resuscitation

C   Close observation

D   Immediate open thoracotomy

E   Insertion of chest drain

F   Needle aspiration

G   Needle thoracocentesis

H   Pericardiocentesis

I   Urgent arteriography

For each of the following scenarios, choose the best therapeutic option from the list above. Each option may be used once, more than once or not at all.

○   92   A 31-year-old is brought to A&E unconscious. He has been involved in a road traffic accident (RTA). He had a right tension pneumothorax which was treated at the scene by needle thoracocentesis. On arrival he has a heart rate of 134 beats/min, a BP of 82/45 mmHg and an RR of 38 breaths/min. On examination he has absent breath sounds and hyper-resonance on the right side of the chest, with tracheal deviation to the left.

○   93   A 29-year-old man was involved in an RTA. He was the front seat passenger. He is complaining of severe chest pain. On examination he is tachycardic, with a heart rate of 104 beats/min, an RR of 20 breaths/min and a BP of 140/68 mmHg. On examination he has slightly reduced air entry on the left base, which is also dull to percussion. The trachea is slightly deviated to the right. Chest X-ray shows a small left haemothorax and a widened mediastinum.

○   94   A 34-year-old is brought in with a stab wound to the right side of his mediastinum. On arrival in the department he is in cardiac arrest. The ECG trace shows pulseless electrical activity.

THEME: CARCINOGENS

A Bronchial carcinoma

B Burkitt's lymphoma

C Carcinoma of the bladder

D Carcinoma of the cervix

E Mucosa-associated lymphoid tissue lymphoma (MALT tumour)

F Hepatocellular carcinoma

G Hodgkin's lymphoma

H Oropharyngeal carcinoma

From the list above, choose the malignancy associated with exposure to the substances/organisms listed below. You may use each option once, more than once or not at all.

O   95   *Schistosoma*

O   96   B-Naphthylamine

O   97   Epstein–Barr virus

O   98   *Helicobacter pylori*

O   99   *Aspergillus* infection

O   100   Betel nuts

THEME: INOTROPES

A Adrenaline (epinephrine)

B Dobutamine

C Dopamine

D Isoprenaline

E Noradrenaline (norepinephrine)

For each of the following statements, choose the most appropriate inotrope from the list above. Each option may be used once, more than once or not at all.

○ 101 The inotrope which has the greatest bronchodilator effect.

○ 102 The inotrope used in cardiac arrest situations to provoke ventricular fibrillation.

○ 103 The inotrope that in a low dose (less than 4 μg/kg per min) can be used to increase glomerular filtration rate and sodium excretion.

○ 104 The inotrope that is used in the treatment of shock to increase total peripheral resistance, causing increase in both systolic and diastolic blood pressure.

THEME: SCROTAL SWELLINGS

A Epididymo-orchitis

B Fournier's gangrene

C Hydrocoele

D Testicular malignancy

E Testicular torsion

F Testicular trauma

G Torsion of hydatid of Morgagni

H Varicocele

For each of the following scenarios, choose the most likely diagnosis from the list above. Each option may be used once, more than once or not at all.

○ 105 A 23-year-old man presents with acute scrotal pain. The right testicle is exquisitely tender and is higher than the left. There is some superficial erythema.

○ 106 A 65-year-old man presents with a scrotal swelling. It has recently enlarged, but is painless. Examination reveals a large soft swelling which transilluminates.

○ 107 A 70-year-old diabetic man presents in septic shock. The scrotum is swollen and dusky purple.

THEME: TRAUMA

A Application of hard collar and head restraints

B Computed tomography (CT) scan of the head

C Full spinal and neurological assessment

D Immobilisation

E Intubation

F Plain X-rays of the skull

For each of the following scenarios, choose the most appropriate next step from the list above. Each option may be used once, more than once or not at all.

○ 108 A 38-year-old man in a hard collar and with head restraints is brought to A&E by the paramedics on a spinal board. He has fallen from a horse. On arrival, he is unconscious and makes no response to painful stimuli. He has a large boggy swelling around his left occiput.

○ 109 A 26-year-old man falls approximately 6 m down from a ladder. He has been unable to walk since, complaining of pain in his feet. X-rays requested from triage confirm bilateral calcaneal fractures.

○ 110 A 48-year-old man is brought to A&E following an RTA. He was unconscious at the scene, but on arrival at the department he was fully conscious. He is now talking in a confused manner, opening his eyes in response to pain, and localising to pain.

THEME: LOCAL ANAESTHETICS

A 5 ml

B 10 ml

C 20 ml

D 30 ml

E 40 ml

F 50 ml

G 60 ml

H 80 ml

What is the maximum volume of each of the local anaesthetic agents given below that can safely be used in an 80-kg man who is otherwise healthy. Each option may be used once, more than once or not at all.

O   111 Lidocaine 2%.

O   112 Bupivacaine 0.5%.

O   113 Bupivacaine 0.25% with 1 in 200 000 adrenaline.

O   114 Lidocaine 1% with 1 in 200 000 adrenaline.

THEME: CHEMOTHERAPY

A Adjuvant chemotherapy

B Neo-adjuvant chemotherapy

C No chemotherapy

For each of the following scenarios, choose the most appropriate option from the list above. Each option may be used once, more than once or not at all.

115 A 46-year-old woman presents with a breast lump. After wide local excision and axillary node clearance she is found to have ductal carcinoma in situ with the excision margins clear and no lymph node involvement.

116 A 54-year-old man has a right hemicolectomy. The histopathological report is well differentiated Duke's B carcinoma with vascular invasion.

117 A 42-year-old woman has a cystectomy for squamous cell carcinoma of the bladder. The histopathological report is a poorly differentiated tumour with micrometastases in adjacent lymph nodes. A pre-operative staging CT did not show any evidence of metastasis.

THEME: DIAGNOSIS OF ENDOCRINE DISORDERS

A 24-hour urinary vanillylmandelic acid (VMA)

B Dexamethasone suppression test

C Plasma aldosterone levels

D Radio-immunoassay of 17-hydroxyprogesterone

E Serum calcitonin

F Short Synacthen test

G Vitamin D levels

For each of the following scenarios, choose the most appropriate investigation from the list above. Each option may be used once, more than once or not at all.

O   118 A 36-year-old man presents with a history of intermittent hypertension, anxiety, palpitations, tachycardia and excess sweating. Phaeochromocytoma is suspected.

O   119 A 46-year-old woman with history of vitiligo and rheumatoid arthritis presents with pigmentation of the buccal mucosa and skin, loss of body hair and postural hypotension, suggestive of Addison's disease.

O   120 A 54-year-old woman presents with hypertension, polyuria and polydipsia. Renal function, blood sugar and calcium levels are all normal. Conn syndrome is suspected.

O   121 A 6-year-old child with short stature, penile enlargement and history of failure to thrive as an infant is suspected of having congenital adrenal hyperplasia.

O   122 A 24-year-old woman is referred for investigation after developing excessive hair growth and acne, purple striae over the abdomen and central obesity.

THEME: TERMS USED FOR DISORDERS OF GROWTH AND DIFFERENTIATION

A Agenesis

B Atrophy

C Dysplasia

D Hyperplasia

E Hypertrophy

F Hypoplasia

G Metaplasia

H Neoplasia

For each of the following descriptions, choose the most appropriate option from the list above. Each option may be used once, more than once or not at all.

O 123 Increased numbers of red blood cells in individuals living at altitude.

O 124 Weakness, reduced size and function of an arm immobilised for a long period of time.

O 125 Change of bladder transitional cell epithelium to squamous epithelium following *Schistosoma haematobium* infection.

O 126 Anencephaly (failure of neural tube development).

THEME: CONDITIONS CAUSED BY MICROBES

A *Candida albicans*

B *Clostridium difficile*

C *Clostridium perfringens*

D *Escherichia coli*

E *Helicobacter pylori*

F *Staphylococcus aureus*

G *Streptococcus faecalis*

H *Streptococcus pyogenes*

For each of the following scenarios, choose the most appropriate option from the list above. Each option may be used once, more than once or not at all.

O 127 A 42-year-old HIV-positive man with white fluffy patches in the mouth surrounded by painful areas of erythema.

O 128 A 12-year-old girl with an enlarging, hot, tender, erythematous area on her right leg which began as an insect bite.

O 129 A 42-year-old diabetic woman with dysuria, frequency and offensive-smelling urine.

O 130 A 66-year-old gentleman who had a recent operation for evacuation of traumatic haematoma of the thigh develops discoloration and swelling at the operation site, with crepitus on examination and a subcutaneous gas collection visible on X-ray.

O 131 An 84-year-old woman, treated for 4 weeks with co-amoxiclav (Augmentin) for a respiratory tract infection, develops profuse, offensive-smelling diarrhoea.

O 132 A 33-year-old man presents to A&E with severe epigastric pain and signs of peritonism. Erect chest X-ray shows air under the diaphragm.

THEME: HYPERSENSITIVITY REACTIONS

A Type I hypersensitivity reaction

B Type II hypersensitivity reaction

C Type III hypersensitivity reaction

D Type IV hypersensitivity reaction

For each of the following scenarios, choose the most appropriate option from the list above. Each option may be used once, more than once or not at all.

○ 133 A 42-year-old woman develops itching, swelling and erythema at the site of the nickel buckle of a new watch.

○ 134 A 15-year-old girl has a streptococcal throat infection, then goes on to develop post-streptococcal glomerulonephritis.

○ 135 A 14-year-old boy develops sneezing and watering of the eyes in the summer months when the pollen count is high.

○ 136 A 44-year-old renal transplant patient develops graft-versus-host disease.

○ 137 A 22-year-old man develops wheezing, rash and swelling of the mouth and tongue after eating a peanut.

○ 138 A baby develops haemolytic disease of the newborn. The mother is rhesus-negative.

THEME: GLASGOW COMA SCALE SCORES

A 4

B 6

C 7

D 8

E 10

F 13

G 14

For each of the following scenarios, choose the most appropriate score from the list above. Each option may be used once, more than once or not at all.

○ 139 A 25-year-old motorcyclist is involved in a head-on collision with a lorry. On arrival in A&E he is unable to obey commands, but localises to pain and is able to speak but appears confused. He only opens his eyes in response to pain.

○ 140 A 66-year-old man has a fall in the street, hitting his head. On initial assessment GCS is 15. However, on arrival in A&E he is unable to obey commands and withdraws only from painful stimuli, making incomprehensible sounds and not opening his eyes at all.

○ 141 A 44-year-old known intravenous drug user (IVDU) is brought to A&E after being found collapsed after a suspected overdose. He will not open his eyes in response to commands but does so in response to painful stimuli. His pupils are pinpoint. His only movement is withdrawal from pain and he doesn't speak.

○ 142 A 29-year-old man involved in a pub brawl is hit over the head with a glass bottle. He is able to give a partial history but appears quite confused. He opens his eyes when spoken to and moves on command.

THEME: MANAGEMENT OF TRANSITIONAL CELL CARCINOMA OF THE BLADDER

A Brachytherapy

B Cystectomy + reconstruction

C Cystectomy + urethrectomy + ileal conduit

D Intravesical chemotherapy

E MVAC chemotherapy

F Nephrectomy

G Nephro-uretectomy

H Transurethral resection of bladder tumour (TURBT)

For each of the following scenarios, choose the most appropriate option from the list above. Each option may be used once, more than once or not at all.

○ 143 A 45-year-old woman presents with a 3-week history of haematuria. An IVU reveals a filling defect in the renal pelvis. This is confirmed as a soft-tissue mass on CT scan.

○ 144 A 55-year-old woman is found to have widespread carcinoma in situ (CIS) on cystoscopy and biopsy. She is treated initially with several instillations of intravesical BCG. Repeat cystoscopy shows no change in the CIS and urethral biopsy confirms CIS. She is keen to have aggressive treatment.

THEME: HAEMORRHAGIC SHOCK

A Class I haemorrhagic shock

B Class II haemorrhagic shock

C Class III haemorrhagic shock

D Class IV haemorrhagic shock

For each of the following scenarios, choose the most appropriate option from the list above. Each option may be used once, more than once or not at all.

145 A 20-year-old man involved in an RTA sustains bilateral fractured femurs. He is brought to A&E, where on assessment he is found to be anxious and confused, with a pulse of 130/min and BP of 70/50 mmHg. Urine output over 1 hour is 10 ml.

146 A 70-year-old patient with a known 5-cm abdominal aortic aneurysm is admitted to A&E with severe central abdominal pain that radiates to the back. Prior to resuscitation, his pulse is 110/min, BP 120/100 mmHg and RR 24 breaths/min. He is slightly anxious but fully lucid.

147 A 60-year-old alcoholic has three episodes of haematemesis (total 500 ml) and melaena. On examination, he is anxious, sweaty and uncooperative with a pulse of 126/min, BP 80/60 mmHg and RR 24 breaths/min.

THEME: MANAGEMENT OF THYROID DISEASE

A　Carbimazole

B　Hemithyroidectomy

C　Propranolol

D　Propylthiouracil

E　Radio-iodine ablation

F　Subtotal thyroidectomy

G　Thyroxine

H　Total thyroidectomy

For each of the following scenarios, choose the most appropriate management option from the list above. Each option may be used once, more than once or not at all.

○　148　A 20-year-old woman presents with a smooth goitre, weight loss, palpitations and diarrhoea. She is diagnosed as having Graves' disease but is unable to tolerate carbimazole due to development of agranulocytosis.

○　149　A 36-year-old woman is in her second trimester of pregnancy. She was mildly thyrotoxic at first but is increasingly symptomatic and requires treatment.

○　150　A 56-year-old woman diagnosed with toxic multinodular goitre which is unresponsive to medical treatment.

○　151　A 54-year-old woman presents with a goitre which has been there for a long time but was not bothering her. She is now having some difficulty breathing when lying down and feels 'pressure' in her throat.

THEME: CAUSES OF JAUNDICE

A Carcinoma of the head of the pancreas

B Gallstones

C Gilbert syndrome

D Haemolytic anaemia

E Hepatitis

F Primary liver carcinoma

For each of the following scenarios, choose the most appropriate diagnosis from the list above. Each option may be used once, more than once or not at all.

○ 152 A 20-year-old woman presents with complaints of dark-coloured urine, pale stools and weight loss for a few weeks. On examination she has painless jaundice.

○ 153 A 10-year-old boy with known sickle cell disease presents with pain in the epigastric region. On examination he has jaundice.

○ 154 A known intravenous drug misuser with a history of hepatitis B presents with jaundice and loss of weight. Blood tests reveal raised α-fetoprotein. He admits sharing needles with other drug misusers.

THEME: KNEE INJURIES

A Anterior cruciate ligament tear

B Lateral meniscus tear

C Medial collateral ligament tear

D Medial meniscus tear

E Patella fracture

F Posterior cruciate ligament tear

For each of the following scenarios, choose the most appropriate option from the list above. Each option may be used once, more than once or not at all.

 155 A 35-year-old rugby player twists his knee during a match. It gradually swells and becomes tender, and he finds himself unable to fully extend it. It is tender over the medial joint line. An X-ray shows evidence of an effusion. Despite aspiration of the traumatic effusion, he is still unable to fully extend the knee.

 156 A 25-year-old footballer hyperextends his knee while attempting to kick the ball. He hears a loud 'popping' sound. The knee swells up immediately. In the following weeks his knee is painful on weight-bearing and gives way without warning.

THEME: TREATMENT OF PROSTATE CANCER

A Androgen ablation

B Brachytherapy

C External beam radiotherapy

D Radical prostatectomy

E Surveillance

For each of the following scenarios, choose the most appropriate option from the list above. Each option may be used once, more than once or not at all.

○ 157 An 80-year-old man diagnosed with a pT_1 prostate cancer, an incidental finding when the chips obtained from TURP were examined.

○ 158 A 50-year-old man with pT_2 prostate cancer diagnosed on rectal biopsy wants curative treatment. He is sexually active and wants to have a minimal chance of developing incontinence and impotence, and wants to reduce the amount of time spent in hospital. He has a small-volume prostate.

○ 159 A 65-year-old man was diagnosed as having prostate cancer with lung and bony metastases and local invasion. He was treated with androgen ablation for 6 months but is now complaining of increasing bony and pelvic pain.

THEME: MANAGEMENT OF ANKLE INJURIES

A Arthrodesis

B Closed reduction and plaster of Paris

C Open reduction and internal fixation

D Strict non-weight-bearing and physiotherapy only

E Support, non-steroidal anti-inflammatory drugs (NSAIDs) and early mobilisation

For each of the following scenarios, choose the most appropriate option from the list above. Each option may be used once, more than once or not at all.

○ 160 A 46-year-old woman stumbles on a pavement kerb, landing awkwardly on her left ankle. She is unable to weight bear. An X-ray shows a fracture of the lateral malleolus only.

○ 161 A 34-year-old footballer has an eversion injury to the right ankle, resulting in an avulsion fracture of the medial malleolus. An X-ray also shows an undisplaced fracture of the fibula at the junction between the middle and lower thirds of the shaft.

○ 162 A 29-year-old woman stumbles while running for the bus, landing heavily on her left ankle. The ankle becomes swollen over the lateral aspect and she has difficulty weight-bearing. An X-ray shows no fracture.

THEME: COMPLICATIONS OF COLORECTAL CANCER

A Appendicitis

B Colocolic intussusception

C Fistula formation

D Haemorrhage

E Invasion into adjacent organ

F Obstruction

For each of the following scenarios, choose the most appropriate option from the list above. Each option may be used once, more than once or not at all.

163 A 69-year-old man presents with a caecal mass presumed to be adenocarcinoma. While undergoing staging investigations, he develops right-sided abdominal pain, guarding and rebound in the right iliac fossa (RIF) associated with fever. There is a mild pyrexia and raised white blood cell count.

164 A 70-year-old man with a known tumour of the transverse colon presents with spasms of abdominal pain, abdominal distension and dehydration. A new sausage-shaped mass is palpable in the epigastrium.

165 A 52-year-old man with metastatic adenocarcinoma of the transverse colon presents with faecal vomiting.

THEME: ABNORMALITIES OF CALCIUM BALANCE

A Addison's disease

B Hypercalcaemia of malignancy

C Hypoparathyroidism

D Primary hyperparathyroidism

E Secondary hyperparathyroidism

F Tertiary hyperparathyroidism

For each of the following scenarios, choose the most appropriate diagnosis from the list above. Each option may be used once, more than once or not at all.

○ 166 A 69-year-old woman presents with paraesthesia, muscle cramps and a tingling sensation around the mouth. She has a past history of thyroidectomy for benign goitre.

○ 167 A 54-year-old renal dialysis patient is found to have raised serum calcium and parathyroid hormone (PTH) levels.

○ 168 A 47-year-old woman with a history of postural hypotension and pigmentation of the buccal mucosa and skin is admitted as an emergency with abdominal pain and constipation. She had an episode of renal colic 2 weeks ago.

THEME: MANAGEMENT OF BENIGN PROSTATIC HYPERPLASIA

A Doxazosin

B Finasteride

C Long-term urethral catheter

D Open prostatectomy

E Suprapubic catheter

F Transurethral incision of prostate

G Transurethral resection of prostate (TURP)

H Trial without catheter (TWOC) and α-blocker

I TWOC alone

For each of the following scenarios, choose the most appropriate option from the list above. Each option may be used once, more than once or not at all.

169 A 60-year-old man, day 1 post-op right shoulder hemiarthroplasty for severe arthritis develops acute urinary retention. He is catheterised and found to have a residual volume of 800 ml. Digital rectal examination (DRE) shows a smooth, benign, moderately sized prostate.

170 A 65-year-old man has bladder outflow obstruction secondary to benign prostatic hyperplasia (BPH) confirmed by urodynamic studies. Initial success with medical management has been followed by worsening of symptoms, severely affecting his quality of life. DRE reveals a benign-feeling prostate, 50 g in size. Transrectal ultrasound shows no hypoechogenic areas. The patient is very fit, well and active and will not accept long-term catheterisation.

171 A 56-year-old man recently remarried and wants to start a family. He has long-standing symptoms of hesitancy, frequency and terminal dribbling. He recently developed occasional haematuria – fully investigated and not found to be due to any other cause than BPH. DRE and ultrasound scan reveal a benign 40-g prostate.

THEME: WOUND COMPLICATIONS

A Abscess

B Delayed healing

C Evisceration

D Incisional hernia

E Superficial infection

F Wound dehiscence

For each of the following scenarios, choose the most appropriate option from the list above. Each option may be used once, more than once or not at all.

O 172 A patient who has undergone appendicectomy has the sutures removed and the medial 2 cm of the wound opens up, with only a small serous discharge.

O 173 A patient who has undergone laparotomy has pink fluid oozing from the wound a day before having the sutures removed. The wound opens and the bowel extrudes.

O 174 A patient who is 5 days post-op following appendicectomy develops low-grade pyrexia. The wound is full and very tender, and pressure on the medial aspect causes pus to extrude.

THEME: MANAGEMENT OF HERNIAS

A Conservative management

B Laparoscopic repair

C Mayo's operation 'vest over pants'

D Mesh repair

E Repair via crural (Lockwood) approach

F Repair via high inguinal (Lotheissen) approach

G Resection of bowel, anatomosis and repair of abdominal wall defect

H Shouldice repair

For each of the following scenarios, choose the most appropriate course of action from the list above. Each option may be used once, more than once or not at all.

○ 175 A 1-year-old infant of African origin has had an umbilical hernia since birth. He is asymptomatic.

○ 176 A 38-year-old man presents to the outpatients department with a femoral hernia which is non-tender and with no evidence of strangulation or obstruction. He wants to have it repaired.

○ 177 A fit and well 32-year-old man develops bilateral inguinal hernias which are increasing in size and becoming unsightly. He has not had any abdominal surgery previously.

THEME: TREATMENT OF URINARY TRACT INFECTIONS

A Aciclovir

B Fluconazole

C Intravenous co-amoxiclav (Augmentin)

D Metronidazole

E Mitomycin

F Oral ciprofloxacin

G Rifampicin

For each of the following scenarios, choose the most appropriate option from the list above. Each option may be used once, more than once or not at all.

178 A 24-year-old woman presents with a several-month history of recurrent urinary tract infections (UTIs), recent night sweats and weight loss. Mid-stream urine shows many white blood cells but fails to grow any bacteria. She spent her childhood in Bangladesh.

179 A 47-year-old diabetic woman presents with dysuria, frequency and urgency. The urine is cloudy and smells offensive and is positive for nitrites and leucocytes on urine dipstick. She is systemically well.

180 A 52-year-old man presents to A&E with a 2-day history of feeling generally unwell. Over the last 12 hours he has developed right loin pain and rigors and has a temperature of 39 °C. Urine dipstick is positive for nitrites.

THEME: POST-OPERATIVE CRITICAL CARE

A Anaphylactic shock

B Cardiogenic shock

C Hypovolaemic shock

D Neurogenic shock

E Septic shock

For each of the following scenarios, choose the most appropriate option from the list above. Each option may be used once, more than once or not at all.

181 A post-operative patient in ICU has a pulse of 112/min, central venous pressure (CVP) 1 mmHg, cardiac output 4 l/min, and stroke volume 50 ml.

182 A post-operative patient in ICU has: pulse 40/min, CVP 4 mmHg, cardiac output 3 l/min, and stroke volume 80 ml.

183 A post-operative patient in ICU has: pulse 109/min, CVP 5 mmHg, cardiac output 6 l/min, and stroke volume 40 ml.

THEME: SKIN LESIONS

A Basal cell carcinoma

B Bowen's disease

C Kaposi's sarcoma

D Keratoacanthoma

E Lentigo maligna

F Malignant melanoma

G Seborrhoeic warts

H Skin tag

I Solar keratosis

J Squamous cell carcinoma

For each of the following scenarios, choose the most likely diagnosis from the list above. Each option may be used once, more than once or not at all.

O 184 A 64-year-old man presents with a circumscribed scaly plaque approximately 4 cm in diameter on the right calf. Histological examination shows full-thickness epidermal dysplasia.

O 185 A 52-year-old man presents with an irregularly pigmented plaque on the left cheek, which has been increasing in size and was initially uniformly pigmented.

O 186 An 84-year-old man presents with an enlarging painless ulcer with everted edges on the back of his neck. It has been bleeding intermittently.

O 187 A 65-year-old woman presents with a 1-month history of an ulcer over the angle of the mandible with a rolled pearly edge.

QUESTIONS
PRACTICE PAPER 2

THEME: WOUND CLOSURE

A Healing by secondary intention with simple dressings

B Primary closure

C Split-thickness skin graft

D Full-thickness skin graft

E Local flap

F Free flap

For each of the following scenarios, choose the most appropriate option from the list above. Each option may be used once, more than once or not at all.

1 A 45-year-old man with a grade IIIA open fracture of the tibia with loss of skin, fascia and muscle, and bone exposed over a 4-cm-diameter area mid-shin. No infection present.

2 A 25-year-old woman with an injury to the pulp of the right middle finger, with a loss of approximately 1 cm of tissue. Bone not exposed, no infection present.

3 A 29-year-old woman undergoing mastectomy for breast cancer, wishing to have a primary reconstruction.

4 A 50-year-old man with a scalp laceration with an area of skin loss and fascia, down to bone, approximately 2 cm in diameter. No infection.

5 Coverage of a 10-cm-diameter area of burns.

6 A 35-year-old man with a degloving injury to the right arm, approximately 6 cm in extent, with the deep fascia still intact. No infection.

THEME: CARDIAC MURMURS

A Mitral stenosis

B Mitral regurgitation

C Aortic stenosis

D Aortic regurgitation

E Atrial septal defect

F Ventricular septal defect

G Patent ductus arteriosus

For each of the following scenarios, choose the correct defect from the list above. Each option may be used once, more than once or not at all.

7 A 74-year-old woman is admitted with a fractured neck of femur. She reports several recent episodes of 'fainting' and increasing shortness of breath on exertion. Her apex beat is undisplaced and an ejection systolic murmur is heard from the base radiating to the carotids, loudest at the second intercostal space to the right of the sternum.

8 A 70-year-old man attending pre-op clinic reports a 1-year history of exertional dyspnoea and palpitations. He has a malar flush, irregular pulse and undisplaced apex beat. A mid-diastolic murmur is heard.

9 A 50-year-old man admitted with right upper quadrant pain reports increasing shortness of breath. He has an irregular pulse, raised JVP and bilateral pitting oedema. The apex beat is undisplaced and a pulmonary ejection systolic murmur is heard.

10 A 4-month-old baby presents with abdominal pain, pneumonia and failure to thrive. He has had several previous chest infections. He has a systolic murmur, loudest in the second intercostal space at the left sternal edge.

11 A 60-year-old woman in the pre-op clinic reports a 6-month history of dyspnoea, associated with palpitations. A water-hammer pulse is felt, and Corrigan's and Quincke's signs are noted. Her apex beat is displaced and a high-pitched early systolic murmur is heard.

THEME: TREATMENT OF TESTICULAR TUMOURS

A Chemotherapy

B Chemotherapy and radiotherapy

C Orchidectomy and prophylactic radiotherapy

D Orchidectomy and surveillance

E Radiotherapy

F Retroperitoneal lymph node dissection

G Testicular biopsy

For each of the following scenarios, choose the most appropriate treatment from the list above. Each option may be used once, more than once or not at all.

12 A 22-year-old man presents with hard swelling of the left testis and undergoes orchidectomy. Histological examination shows non-seminomatous germ cell tumour. Staging CT scan shows retroperitoneal lymphadenopathy but no nodes above the diaphragm.

13 A 30-year-old man with right-sided undescended testis develops a mass in the left testicle. Left orchidectomy shows seminoma. CT scan shows no evidence of spread.

14 A 35-year-old man develops a hard right testicular mass. He undergoes orchidectomy, which shows it to be a seminoma. A staging CT scan shows lymph node spread above and below the diaphragm.

THEME: TYPES OF HERNIA

A Direct inguinal hernia

B Femoral hernia

C Indirect inguinal hernia

D Littre's hernia

E Lumbar hernia

F Paraumbilical hernia

G Spigelian hernia

H Maydl's hernia

I Epigastric hernia

J Richter's hernia

K Umbilical hernia

For each of the following scenarios, choose the most appropriate option from the list above. Each option may be used once, more than once or not at all.

15 A 58-year-old man with previous laparotomy for diverticular disease develops a hernia at the lower end of his midline scar. The hernia becomes irreducible and he presents to A&E with severe pain. At operation the contents of the hernia show a strangulated Meckel's diverticulum.

16 A 52-year-old woman presents with a tender swelling in the left groin. Examination reveals that this is irreducible with a cough impulse, and lies below and lateral to the pubic tubercle.

17 A 28-year-old man presents with a groin swelling, which is easily reducible and has a cough impulse. On standing, the hernia descends into the scrotum. Reducing the hernia and placing pressure 1 cm above the midpoint of the inguinal ligament prevents the hernia from reappearing.

O 18 A 78-year-old man presents with a reducible mass just superior to the right iliac crest.

O 19 A 78-year-old man with a past history of chronic obstructive pulmonary disease (COPD) presents with a swelling that is protruding through the linea alba, adjacent to the umbilical cicatrix.

O 20 A 44-year-old woman with a 3-month history of an aching lump is seen in clinic. There is a swelling protruding through the bands of the internal oblique at the level of the line of Douglas.

O 21 A 52-year-old man presents with a painful, irreducible lump, which contains the antimesenteric border of the bowel.

THEME: BONE TUMOURS

A Angiosarcoma

B Chondrosarcoma

C Ewing's sarcoma

D Giant-cell tumour

E Metastasis from lung carcinoma

F Myeloma

G Osteoblastoma

H Osteosarcoma

For each of the following scenarios, choose the most likely diagnosis from the list above. Each option may be used once, more than once or not at all.

○ 22 A 15-year-old boy presents with a painful enlarging mass of the lower left femur. An X-ray shows a sclerotic lesion with periosteal elevation. The knee joint is not involved. Chest X-ray shows lesions suspicious of pulmonary metastases. He has a past medical history of retinoblastoma as a child.

○ 23 A 60-year-old gentleman with a past history of multiple osteochondromas affecting the right proximal humerus and ribs presents with a slowly enlarging mass of the right humerus. The X-ray shows endosteal scalloping and cortical thickening. There is evidence of pulmonary spread on chest X-ray.

○ 24 A 10-year-old girl presents with a tender enlarging mass affecting the diaphysis of the left femur. An X-ray shows this to be a lytic lesion. Biopsy identifies it as being a tumour of vascular endothelium.

○ 25 An 80-year-old man with known Paget's disease affecting both legs presents with a painful mass affecting the right tibia. An X-ray shows a lytic lesion arising from the medullary cavity. Pulmonary metastases are present on chest X-ray.

THEME: MANAGEMENT OF ACUTE ISCHAEMIA

A Amputation

B Angioplasty

C Embolectomy

D Management of risk factors

E Reconstruction

F Thrombolysis

G Watch and wait

For each of the following scenarios, choose the most appropriate option from the list above. Each option may be used once, more than once or not at all.

26 A 72-year-old man has history of atrial fibrillation but not of peripheral vascular disease or claudication pain. He presents to A&E with a 2-hour history of an acutely ischaemic left leg. Angiography shows a blockage at the origin of the left femoral artery.

27 An 84-year-old woman, who lives alone, presents with a 36-hour history of acute ischaemia of right foot. Angiography shows occlusion of the right superficial femoral artery.

28 A 64-year-old man, a heavy smoker, has a history of intermittent claudication affecting the right calf. He presents with an acutely ischaemic right leg. On examination the limb is found to be insensate. Angiography shows occlusion of the right femoral artery with good distal run-off.

29 A 70-year-old woman has a history of acute on chronic ischaemic right leg. This was treated initially with thrombolysis, which failed. An angiogram shows occlusion of the superficial femoral artery with poor distal run-off.

THEME: NECK LUMPS

A Branchial cyst

B Cystic hygroma

C Lymph node

D Lymphoma

E Thyroglossal cyst

F Thyroid carcinoma

G Toxic multinodular goitre

H Cervical rib

I Pharyngeal pouch

J Chemodectoma

For each of the following scenarios, choose the most appropriate diagnosis from the list above. Each option may be used once, more than once or not at all.

30 A 12-year-old child presents with a painless midline neck swelling which is fluctuant on palpation. It moves both on swallowing and on protrusion of the tongue.

31 A 2-year-old boy presents with unilateral painless swelling at the base of the neck. It brilliantly transilluminates.

32 A 25-year-old woman presents with an irregular, painless, midline neck swelling which moves on swallowing but not on protrusion of the tongue. She also complains of feeling anxious and sweaty, and has lost some weight in recent weeks.

33 A 35-year-old man presents with an enlarging neck lump between the junction of the upper and middle thirds of the anterior border of the left sternocleidomastoid muscle. The mass is non-tender.

O   34   A 69-year-old gentleman presents with weight loss, epigastric pain and a hard lump in the supraclavicular fossa.

O   35   A 50-year-old man attends complaining of a painless lump in the neck. On examination a 4-cm, smooth, firm lump is found in the upper part of the anterior triangle of the neck. It is pulsatile and, on further questioning, the patient admits to a number of recent blackouts.

THEME: SURGICAL MANAGEMENT OF INFLAMMATORY BOWEL DISEASE

A Colectomy and ileorectal anastomosis

B Extended right hemicolectomy

C Ileo-caecal resection

D Proctocolectomy and ileo-anal pouch

E Proctocolectomy and ileostomy

F Stricturoplasty

G Subtotal colectomy + ileostomy + mucous fistula

For each of the following scenarios, choose the most appropriate option from the list above. Each option may be used once, more than once or not at all.

○ **36** A 15-year-old boy with a history of ulcerative colitis for 5 years has a 2-year history of severe disease, resulting in weight loss and growth failure. He is commenced on increasing doses of steroids without success. Disease is present from transverse colon to rectum.

○ **37** A 39-year-old gentleman with ulcerative colitis presents with a severe acute exacerbation. Three days after admission he develops severe abdominal pain, becomes septic, and on examination has a rigid abdomen with peritonism. Erect chest X-ray shows air under the diaphragm.

○ **38** A 27-year-old woman with Crohn's disease is admitted for the fourth occasion in 6 months with small-bowel obstruction. Barium follow-through shows a 4-cm stricture of the proximal ileum.

○ 39 A 22-year-old woman with diagnosis of Crohn's disease has a history over the past year of recurrent anaemia and weight loss. Colonoscopy shows severe inflammation and active disease affecting the caecum and terminal ileum. Maximum medical therapy has been unsuccessful.

○ 40 A 21-year-old patient with a history of severe ulcerative colitis has failed on medical treatment alone. Investigations show rectal sparing.

THEME: SCROTAL SWELLINGS

A Acute epididymo-orchitis

B Encysted hydrocoele of the cord

C Epididymal cyst

D Chronic epididymo-orchitis

E Haematocele

F Hydrocoele

G Inguino-scrotal hernia

H Sebaceous cyst

I Testicular tumour

J Varicocele

For each of the following scenarios, choose the most appropriate option from the list above. Each option may be used once, more than once or not at all.

41 A 42-year-old man presents with a non-tender right scrotal swelling which has been gradually increasing in size over several months. On examination it is fluctuant and transilluminates. It is not possible to feel the right testicle separately from the swelling, but it is possible to get above it and feel the cord as a separate structure.

42 A 65-year-old man presents with a slowly enlarging painless scrotal swelling. On examination it is fluctuant and transilluminates. It is possible to get above it on examination and feel the testis as a separate structure. The swelling is found to lie above and slightly behind the testis.

43 A 70-year-old man has a history of a long-standing 'aching' sensation in the right testis. On examination he has a firm craggy mass and a few discharging sinuses on the scrotal skin. Urine microscopy shows sterile pyuria.

44 A 38-year-old man presents with a left-sided scrotal swelling. On examination it is a soft, compressible swelling which does not have a cough impulse. It is not possible to get above it and it disappears on lying down.

45 A 45-year-old man presents with a right-sided scrotal swelling which increases in size on standing up. On examination it is not transilluminable and it is not possible to get above it. There is a positive cough impulse.

46 A 25-year-old man presents with a smooth, left-sided, painless scrotal swelling which is transilluminable and fluctuant. It is possible to feel the testis as a separate structure below the swelling.

THEME: UPPER LIMB FRACTURES

A Barton's fracture

B Bennett's fracture

C Colles' fracture

D Galeazzi's fracture

E Monteggia's fracture

F Smith's fracture

For each of the following scenarios, choose the most appropriate option from the list above. Each option may be used once, more than once or not at all.

47 A 24-year-old woman presents with a painful left arm following an RTA. The X-ray shows a fracture of the upper third of the ulna together with an associated dislocated radial head.

48 An 84-year-old woman has a fall in the street, landing on her right hand, which appears swollen and deformed. An X-ray shows a fracture of the distal radius, which is angulated dorsally. The fracture extends intra-articularly and there is subluxation of the carpus.

49 A 76-year-old woman stumbles down the stairs at home, landing heavily on her left arm. On examination she has a deformed, bruised left wrist. An X-ray shows an extra-articular fracture of the distal radius, which is displaced volarly.

50 A 15-year-old boy is knocked off his bicycle and lands on his right arm. He presents to A&E with a swollen tender wrist. An X-ray shows a fracture of the mid-shaft of the radius and dislocation of the inferior radio-ulnar joint.

THEME: STAGING OF COLON CANCER

A Duke's A stage

B Duke's B stage

C Duke's C stage

D Duke's D stage

For each of the following clinical scenarios, select the most appropriate stage. Each answer may be used once, more than once or not at all.

51   A 68-year-old man presents with weight loss and iron-deficiency anaemia. Colonoscopy confirms a caecal mass. The specimen obtained at laparotomy shows adenocarcinoma extending through the bowel wall. All of the nine lymph nodes removed are involved.

52   A 52-year-old man presents with a history of increasingly severe constipation and rectal bleeding. He is found to have a stenosing lesion of the distal sigmoid colon. Biopsy confirms adenocarcinoma. He undergoes anterior resection and the specimen shows three out of the total seven nodes removed are involved.

53   A 25-year-old man from a family known to carry the *HNPCC* gene is found to have a lesion in the transverse colon at colonoscopy. Resection and histological examination of the specimen shows this to be invading the muscle layer of the bowel wall.

THEME: URINARY SYSTEM TRAUMA

A Catheterisation and contrast

B CT scan

C Cystogram

D Retrograde uteropyelography

E Surgical exploration

F Urethrogram

For each of the following scenarios, choose the most appropriate investigation from the list above. Each option may be used once, more than once or not at all.

54 A 25-year-old man slips while walking along the top of a metal gate and falls, straddling the gate. On examination he is in significant pain and has butterfly pattern bruising to the perineum. There is fresh blood at the urethral meatus.

55 A 30-year-old man involved in a fight sustains a blow to the groin with a blunt instrument. On examination there is gross swelling and bruising with an area of tense swelling around the left testicle, which is becoming increasingly large and painful.

56 A 52-year-old man is mugged and stabbed with a knife in the area of the left renal angle. He complains of loin pain. Dipstick shows microscopic haematuria.

THEME: PREPARATION OF PATIENTS FOR ENDOCRINE SURGERY

A Bowel preparation

B Calcitonin infusion

C Corticosteroids

D Phenoxybenzamine and propranolol

E Thallium technetium scan

F Thyroxine

G Vocal cord examination

For each of the following scenarios, choose the most appropriate option from the list above. Each option may be used once, more than once or not at all.

57 A 28-year-old woman with Graves' disease resistant to medical treatment is due to have a subtotal thyroidectomy for symptoms of compression.

58 A 42-year-old patient is planned to have a parathyroidectomy after presenting with raised calcium and parathyroid hormone levels with no history of renal disease.

59 A 34-year-old patient is found to have bilateral adrenal masses on CT, and suspected to have phaeochromocytoma. An adrenalectomy is planned.

THEME: MANAGEMENT OF PAEDIATRIC DISORDERS

A   Broad-spectrum antibiotics

B   Gastrografin enema

C   Laparotomy and duodenostomy

D   Laparotomy and proceed

E   Pneumatic reduction

F   Ramstedt's pyloromyotomy

For each of the following scenarios, choose the most appropriate management option from the list above. Each option may be used once, more than once or not at all.

60   A 40-day-old baby develops projectile vomiting approximately 20 minutes after each feed together with failure to thrive. On examination an olive-shaped mass is noted in the RUQ following feeding. Bloods show a metabolic alkalosis.

61   A 2-day-old baby known to have cystic fibrosis presents with a distended abdomen and bilious vomiting. His rectum is empty.

62   A 1-year-old infant presents with intermittent spasms of abdominal pain associated with drawing up of the legs and a small amount of rectal bleeding. A sausage-shaped mass is noted in the epigastrium. Two similar episodes in the past were treated with hydrostatic reduction.

THEME: RENAL STONES

A   Watch and wait

B   Extracorporeal shock-wave lithotripsy (ESWL)

C   Flexible ureteroscopy

D   Rigid ureteroscopy

E   Laparoscopic ureterolithotomy

F   Percutaneous nephrolithotomy (PCNL)

G   Nephrectomy

For each of the following scenarios, choose the most appropriate management option from the list above. Each option may be used once, more than once or not at all.

63   A 54-year-old woman with a history of renal stone disease presents with a 2-month history of intermittent left loin pain. An intravenous urogram (IVU) shows a 1.5-cm stone in the left renal pelvis but no evidence of obstruction. She has a past history of ischaemic heart disease and has a 4-cm aortic aneurysm lying close to the origin of the left renal artery; this is under surveillance.

64   A 27-year-old man presents to A&E with severe right loin and groin pain and microscopic haematuria on dipstick. Pain is well controlled with NSAIDs and pethidine. An IVU confirms the presence of a 4-mm stone in the right mid-ureter region.

65   A 42-year-old man presents to A&E with severe right loin pain radiating to the groin. He is sweating profusely and vomiting, with a temperature of 38.9 °C. Dipstick shows 3+ blood and 3+ leucocytes. An IVU shows a 5-mm stone in the upper right ureter and dilated calyces.

66   A 24-year-old woman develops severe loin pain with one episode of frank haematuria. She is apyrexial. An IVU shows a 1-cm calculus lying in the lower pole of the right kidney.

O   67   An asymptomatic 29-year-old woman undergoes an ultrasound scan which reveals a 1-cm renal calculus within a cyst.

O   68   A 35-year-old man with right loin to groin pain, who is apyrexial, has a 5-mm calculus in the proximal ureter on IVU.

O   69   A 53-year-old man presents with left loin to groin pain and haematuria. IVU reveals a 1-cm calculus in the lower pole of the right kidney.

THEME: MANAGEMENT OF THYROID CANCER

A Chemotherapy alone

B Lobectomy

C Subtotal thyroidectomy

D Surgery and external beam radiotherapy

E Total thyroidectomy and thyroxine replacement

For each of the following scenarios, choose the most appropriate treatment option from the list above. Each option may be used once, more than once or not at all.

○ 70 A 27-year-old man with history of previous neck irradiation for lymphoma presents with thyroid mass. Fine-needle aspiration reveals cells with 'orphan Annie' nuclei. CT shows localised disease.

○ 71 A 90-year-old woman presents with a hard thyroid mass and a progressively hoarse voice. Cervical lymph nodes are hard and enlarged.

○ 72 A 48-year-old patient with a family history of multiple endocrine neoplasia (MEN) syndrome presents with a thyroid mass that appears malignant but shows no evidence of spread.

○ 73 A 57-year-old woman presents with painless thyroid swelling and weight loss. Fine-needle aspiration of the swelling indicates that it is a lymphoma.

THEME: PRURITUS ANI

A Anal carcinoma

B Anal fissure

C Anal polyp

D Fistula in ano

E Gonorrhoea

F Haemorrhoids

G Syphilis

H Yeast infection

For each of the following scenarios, choose the most appropriate option from the list above. Each option may be used once, more than once or not at all.

74 A 35-year-old woman who regularly takes codeine-based analgesics for tension headaches presents with pruritus ani, rectal bleeding and severe pain following defecation.

75 A 57-year-old HIV-positive man has a history of long-standing anal intra-epithelial neoplasia (AIN) but was lost to follow-up for the past 5 years. He now presents with pruritus ani and a firm ulcerated mass at the anal margin with palpable lymph nodes.

76 A 25-year-old woman with a history of ulcerative colitis on maximum medical therapy to help control disease presents with pruritus ani. On examination the peri-anal area is red, inflamed and excoriated with a well-demarcated edge.

77 A 48-year-old man presents with a 3-month history of weight loss and intermittent fever. He also complains of itching around the anus, associated with soreness and purulent discharge.

THEME: MANAGEMENT OF VENOUS DISEASE OF THE LOWER LIMB

A Debridement and compression bandaging

B Elevation and NSAIDs

C Injection sclerotherapy

D Sapheno-femoral ligation

E Split-skin graft

F Stab avulsions

G Systemic antibiotics

H Topical antibiotics

For each of the following scenarios, choose the most appropriate option from the list above. Each option may be used once, more than once or not at all.

78 A 46-year-old woman has long-standing varicose veins affecting both legs which have recently started to ache. Doppler examination shows no problem with the deep venous system. Varicosities are in the distribution of the long saphenous vein.

79 A 69-year-old woman has a history of deep vein thrombosis affecting the right leg 20 years ago. She now presents with long-standing ulcers over the right gaiter region. ABPI of both legs = 0.8. She is treated with debridement and compression dressing, but review at 12 weeks shows no improvement.

80 An 84-year-old woman with a long-standing venous ulcer of the left shin, treated with regular debridement and dressings, notices it is becoming increasingly tender. On examination the ulcer has a small amount of purulent, offensive discharge and there is surrounding cellulitis.

81 A 60-year-old woman with a 10-year history of varicose veins affecting both legs presents with an acute episode of painful thrombophlebitis.

THEME: ABDOMINAL SIGNS

A Battle's sign

B Boas' sign

C Cullen's sign

D Grey Turner's sign

E Murphy's sign

F Psoas stretch sign

G Rovsing's sign

For each of the following clinical scenarios, choose the most appropriate sign from the list above. Each answer may be used once, more than once or not at all.

○ **82** A 39-year-old man presents to A&E with severe epigastric and RUQ pain radiating through to the back, associated with nausea and vomiting. Inspection of the abdomen shows bruising around the umbilicus.

○ **83** A 54-year-old alcoholic is found collapsed at home in a state of shock. She is unable to give a history but shouts out when her abdomen is palpated. Amylase is 3000 Somogyi U/dl, erect chest X-ray normal. A bluish discoloration is noticed around the flanks.

○ **84** A 45-year-old woman with known gallstones presents with RUQ pain and fever and is found to have a raised WCC. On palpation of the abdomen she is found to be tender in the RUQ and this increases when she breathes in, such that it causes her to stop inspiring.

○ **85** A 27-year-old man presents with right iliac fossa (RIF) pain, preceded by 2 days of generalised abdominal pain and associated vomiting. His WCC is raised. Palpation in the left iliac fossa (LIF) reproduces the pain in the RIF.

THEME: ABDOMINAL INCISIONS

A Gridiron incision

B Kocher's incision

C Lanz incision

D Laparoscopic port incisions

E Midline incision

F Paramedian incision

G Pfannenstiel's incision

H Rooftop incision

I Rutherford–Morrison incision

For each of the following clinical scenarios, choose the most appropriate incision. Each option may be used once, more than once or not at all.

86 A 36-year-old woman presents with abdominal distension. A CT scan reveals a benign-looking right ovarian cyst, 5 × 5 cm. An elective excision is planned.

87 A 38-year-old alcoholic presents with severe epigastric pain. Examination reveals a rigid abdomen and no bowel sounds. Erect chest X-ray shows air under the diaphragm.

88 A 38-year-old woman who is in the second trimester of pregnancy has had multiple episodes of cholecystitis in recent months which are becoming increasingly frequent. She is to have cholecystectomy as soon as possible.

89 A 16-year-old girl presents with central abdominal pain which shifts to the right iliac fossa and is associated with nausea and diarrhoea. She has a low-grade temperature and WCC of 18×10^9/l. Examination reveals rebound tenderness and guarding in the RIF.

90 A 48-year-old woman admitted for curative surgery for carcinoma of the head of the pancreas.

THEME: FULL BLOOD COUNT

Normal values: haemoglobin (Hb) 11.5–16.5 g/dl (women), 13–18 g/dl (men); mean corpuscular volume (MCV) 78–98 fl; white cell count (WCC) 4–11 $\times$ 10^9/l; neutrophils 2.0–7.5 $\times$ 10^9/l; eosinophils 0.05–0.35 $\times$ 10^9/l; platelets 150–400 $\times$ 10^9/l.

Table 2

	Hb	MCV	WCC	Neutrophils	Eosinophils	Platelets
A	10.0	120	9.0	6.0	0.1	300
B	7.0	80	8.0	5.0	0.2	250
C	6.0	60	7.0	4.0	0.1	170
D	13.5	90	19.0	16.0	0.1	290
E	22.0	87	5.0	2.5	0.3	350
F	15.0	89	14.0	7.5	4.0	350

For each of the following scenarios, choose the most appropriate full blood count (FBC) result from the table above. Each option may be used once, more than once or not at all.

○ 91 An 18-year-old girl returns from a gap year in Africa with fever, abdominal pain and diarrhoea. Positive stool sample indicates amoebic dysentery.

○ 92 A 67-year-old chronic alcoholic.

○ 93 A 55-year-old woman on intravenous steroid therapy.

○ 94 A 66-year-old man diagnosed with a friable tumour in the right colon on colonoscopy.

○ 95 A 33-year-old man known to have hereditary elliptocytosis (haemolytic anaemia).

○ 96 A 75-year-old hypertensive man with a diagnosis of polycythaemia rubra vera.

THEME: SALIVARY GLANDS

A Parotid gland

B Sublingual gland

C Submandibular gland

For each of the following scenarios, choose the most appropriate gland from the list above. Each answer may be used once, more than once or not at all.

○ 97 The facial nerve runs through this gland and its blood supply comes from a branch of the external carotid artery. Of tumours arising in this gland, 80% are benign.

○ 98 This gland secretes mucous and serous saliva. Secretomotor fibres come from the parasympathetic system which hitch-hike along with the chorda tympani and lingual nerve.

○ 99 This gland is divided into deep and superficial parts by the posterior border of the mylohyoid muscle. Blood supply comes from the facial artery and vein.

THEME: MANAGEMENT OF HERNIAS

A Conservative management

B Elective hernia repair

C Emergency hernia repair

D Urgent hernia repairs, ie on an elective list but prioritised over benign conditions

For each of the following scenarios, choose the most appropriate course of action from the list above. Each option may be used once, more than once or not at all.

○ 100 A 79-year-old woman presents to clinic with a small (3 cm) non-tender lump in her groin. It has been present for the past 2 months. It lies below and lateral to the pubic tubercle. It is irreducible and there is no cough impulse.

○ 101 A 1-year-old boy presents with a small indirect inguinal hernia.

○ 102 A 65-year-old man presents with an indirect inguinal hernia. It is non-tender and has been present for 3 weeks. It initially reduced spontaneously, but over the past 2 days it has not been reducible.

○ 103 An 84-year-old man with chronic bronchitis, diabetes mellitus and a past medical history of two episodes of myocardial infarction presents with an inguinal hernia. It has been present for 7 years, but for the past day it has been very painful and irreducible. On examination it is tender and erythematous and there is no cough impulse.

○ 104 A healthy 84-year-old man presents to clinic with a small right inguinal hernia. On examination there is a 2-cm-diameter direct hernia which is palpable only on coughing.

○ 105 A 20-year-old man presents with a painless, reducible lump in the right groin, above and medial to the pubic tubercle, extending into the scrotum, which can be controlled with occlusion of the deep inguinal ring.

THEME: STATISTICS

A 4%

B 5%

C 10%

D 20%

E 24%

F 25%

G 75%

H 76%

I 80%

J 90%

K 95%

L 96%

A new test is developed for detecting *Chlamydia*. In a trial 200 people are tested. The test produces 100 positive results and 100 negative results. Of the 100 positive results, 4 are false positives. Of the 100 negative results, 24 are false negatives. From the list above, choose the option to the nearest per cent. You may use each option once, more than once or not at all.

What is the:

O 106 Specificity

O 107 Sensitivity

O 108 Negative predictive value (NPV)

O 109 Positive predictive value (PPV)

THEME: PANCREATIC TUMOURS

A Gastrinoma

B Glucagonoma

C Insulinoma

D Somatostatinoma

E VIPoma

F Carcinoma

G Cystadenocarcinoma

H Cystadenoma

I Zollinger–Ellison tumour

For each of the following scenarios, choose the most likely tumour from the list above. Each option may be used once, more than once or not at all.

○ 110 A 43-year-old man with known parathyroid adenoma presents to A&E with haematemesis.

○ 111 A 64-year-old woman presents with obstructive jaundice and RUQ pain. A random blood glucose is 15.4 mmol/l and an ultrasound scan of the abdomen reveals gallstones.

○ 112 A 50-year-old man with a history of weight loss is found to have a mass on his pancreas on CT. He is discovered to be diabetic. He also has a persistent eczematous rash on his buttocks which has been present for over a year.

○ 113 A 40-year-old woman presents with a 1-year history of epigastric pain. She is prompted to visit A&E following an episode of melaena. Endoscopy reveals multiple peptic ulcers. A CT scan shows tumours affecting the pancreas and duodenum.

○ 114 A 28-year-old man is taken to his GP by his partner, who says he has been behaving strangely and has had eposodes of altered consciousness. This occurs particularly if he skips meals. He has a family history of MEN I.

THEME: BREAST INVESTIGATIONS

A Core biopsy

B CT scan

C Fine-needle aspiration

D Magnetic resonance imaging (MRI)

E No further investigation

F Ultrasound-guided fine-needle aspiration

G Ultrasound scan

For each of the following scenarios, choose the most appropriate investigation from the list above. Each option may be used once, more than once or not at all.

115 A 28-year-old woman presents with a right-sided breast lump. It measures 1 cm in diameter, is mobile, smooth, non-tender, and is superficial to the pectoralis major. There are no associated skin changes. Both axillae are clear. An ultrasound scan is reported as showing a benign lump.

116 A 55-year-old woman is sent to your clinic after screening mammography reveals a suspicious area in the left breast. Clinical examination does not reveal any suspicious areas.

THEME: INTRAVENOUS FLUIDS

A 0.45% Sodium chloride solution

B 0.9% Sodium chloride solution

C 4% Dextrose/0.18% sodium chloride solution

D 5% Dextrose solution

E Compound sodium lactate solution

F Dextran 70

For each of the following questions, choose the most appropriate fluid from the list above. Each option may be used once, more than once or not at all.

O 117 Which fluid has been shown to reduce the incidence of deep venous thrombosis?

O 118 Which fluid is recommended in the Advanced Trauma Life Support (ATLS) guidelines for the initial resuscitation of the trauma patient?

O 119 Which fluid contains 5 mmol of potassium per litre?

O 120 Which fluid contains 150 mmol of sodium per litre?

O 121 Which fluid given in equal volumes expands the intravascular compartment least?

THEME: SPECIFIC TESTS

A Allen's test

B Froment's test

C Lachman's test

D Pivot shift test

E Simmonds' test

F Tinel's test

G Trendelenburg's test

Which test would give the most appropriate information in the following scenarios? Each option may be used once, more than once or not at all.

○ 122 A 21-year-old, very anxious footballer presents to the fracture clinic with an acute swelling of the right knee following a twisting injury 2 days ago. There is no bony tenderness around the knee joint. He is able to fully weight-bear, fully extend his knee and flex to 90 degrees. Aspiration confirms a haemarthrosis.

○ 123 A 69-year-old woman attends the outpatients clinic. On examination she has guttering in the dorsal aspect of her right hand and apparent wasting of the muscles of the hand.

○ 124 A 35-year-old man attends A&E with acute, severe pain in the right calf. He finds it difficult to walk, and cannot plantar-flex his right foot.

THEME: CALCULI

A Bile pigment stone

B Calcium oxalate

C Calcium phosphate

D Cholesterol stone

E Cystine stone

F Urate

For each of the following scenarios, choose the most likely substance for stone formation from the list above. Each option may be used once, more than once or not at all.

○ 125 A 32-year-old man presents with haematuria. A KUB X-ray reveals a staghorn calculus in the right kidney and a mid-stream urine sample grows *proteus*.

○ 126 A 31-year-old woman with known sickle cell anaemia attends A&E with biliary colic. X-rays show the presence of stones in the gallbladder.

○ 127 A 28-year-old man presents with ureteric colic. A KUB study shows a stone at the right vesico-ureteric junction.

THEME: TYPES OF ULCER

A Arterial ulcer

B Curling's ulcer

C Cushing's ulcer

D Duodenal ulcer

E Gastric ulcer

F Marjolin's ulcer

G Rodent ulcer

H Venous ulcer

For each of the following scenarios, choose the most appropriate ulcer from the list above. Each option may be used once, more than once or not at all.

128 A 43-year-old man is admitted to the ICU following an RTA. He has been unconscious and intubated since having a subdural haematoma evacuated. On day 4 of his admission he begins to have blood aspirated from his nasogastric tube.

129 A 76-year-old woman presents to clinic with a large ulcer over her medial malleolus. She has recently noticed that it has grown and bleeds more easily. On examination it has a friable centre and raised edges.

130 An 84-year-old man presents with a small ulcer on the bridge of his nose. It has been present for a number of months. On examination it has pearly white, rolled edges.

131 A 24-year-old has 24% third-degree burns. Three days after his admission he complains of melaena.

THEME: SKIN LESIONS

A Basal cell carcinoma

B Dermatofibroma

C Keratoacanthoma

D Melanoma

E Pyoderma gangrenosum

F Pyogenic granuloma

G Squamous cell carcinoma

H Strawberry naevus

For each of the following scenarios, choose the most likely diagnosis from the list above. Each option may be used once, more than once or not at all.

O 132 A 40-year-old woman presents with a lump on the anterior aspect of the leg. It has been slowly growing over the past 3 years and is now causing cosmetic disfigurement. On examination you find a 1-cm-smooth, firm disc.

O 133 A 2-year-old child is brought to clinic with a small 1-cm lump in her hairline. The lump has been present since birth, but recently it has begun to bleed. On examination the lump is sessile, dark red and has a small ulcerated area in its centre.

O 134 A 76-year-old woman presents with a lesion on her left cheek. There is a small ulcer with a raised pearly edge. She reports that it has been scabbing over, with the scab falling off every now and then.

O 135 A 31-year-old man presents with a mole on his right shoulder. It has grown over the past 2 months and is very itchy. It bleeds occasionally. On examination there is a 2-cm, irregular mole on the shoulder with a surrounding brown halo. He is also jaundiced.

136 A 28-year-old man presents with a lump on the dorsum of his left hand. The lump has grown rapidly over the past 2 weeks. It bleeds easily and is discharging serous fluid. He gives a history of minor trauma to the same hand 3 weeks before. The lump is not painful. On examination there is a bright-red, soft, 1-cm hemispherical lump present.

137 A 64-year-old woman presents with a non-painful lump on her left arm. It has grown rapidly over the past 2 weeks. On examination it is approximately 2 cm in diameter and has a central brown core. It is firm in consistency, but the central core is hard.

THEME: AIRWAY MANAGEMENT

A Bag-valve-mask

B Double-lumen cuffed endotracheal tube

C Nasopharyngeal airway

D Needle cricothyroidotomy

E Oropharyngeal airway

F Percutaneous tracheostomy

G Single-lumen cuffed endotracheal tube

H Single-lumen uncuffed endotracheal tube

For each of the situations below, choose the most appropriate airway adjunct from the list above. Each option may be used once, more than once or not at all.

O **138** A 7-year-old child is brought in to A&E having been rescued from a house fire. He is in respiratory distress and there is evidence of soot around his nasal passages.

O **139** A 64-year-old man due to undergo elective repair of a thoracic aortic aneurysm.

O **140** You are the only doctor in the A&E department. A patient with severe facial injuries suffered in an RTA is brought in by paramedics. He goes into respiratory arrest and an initial attempt at endotracheal intubation fails.

O **141** A 76-year-old man is on the ICU following emergency laparotomy. He is expected to remain there for another week.

O **142** A 27-year-old man involved in a house fire is brought to A&E. He has some singeing of his nasal hair. His RR is 28 breaths/min, and pulse oximetry gives a reading of 94% on 4 l/min oxygen.

THEME: COLORECTAL CARCINOMA PROCEDURES

A Abdomino-perineal resection

B Anterior resection

C Delorme's procedure

D Extended right hemicolectomy

E Hartmann's procedure

F Right hemicolectomy

G Sigmoid colectomy

For each of the following situations, choose the most appropriate operation from the list above. Each option may be used once, more than once or not at all.

○ 143 A patient with carcinoma of the sigmoid colon presenting with peritonitis due to a perforation.

○ 144 A 68-year-old man presents with rectal bleeding. Colonoscopy reveals a caecal tumour.

○ 145 A 76-year-old woman presents with rectal bleeding. Digital rectal examination reveals a tumour 2 cm from the anal margin. This is confirmed by proctoscopy.

○ 146 A 54-year-old woman presents with acute appendicitis. A tumour is found in the appendix at appendicectomy.

○ 147 A 64-year-old man presents with small-bowel obstruction. He gives a 2-month history of a weight loss of 12 kg (2 stone) and intermittent rectal bleeding.

○ 148 An 88-year-old man is found to have a 2-cm tumour of the sigmoid colon. His past medical history includes diabetes mellitus, two episodes of myocardial infarction and peripheral vascular disease.

149 A 77-year-old woman presents with a tumour of the transverse colon, 2 cm from the splenic flexure, which is not causing obstruction; there are no metastases.

150 A 45-year-old man with a non-obtructing tumour of the sigmoid colon without metastases.

151 A 66-year-old man presents with altered bowel habit and he is found to have a tumour approximately 12 cm from the anus. There is no obstruction and there are no metastases.

THEME: THE LIMPING CHILD

A Developmental dysplasia of the hip (DDH)

B Irritable hip

C Osteomyelitis

D Perthes' disease

E Septic arthritis

F Slipped upper femoral epiphysis (SUFE)

G Tuberculosis

For each of the following scenarios, choose the most likely diagnosis from the list above. Each option may be used once, more than once or not at all.

O   152   A 4-year-old boy presents with a sudden-onset limp. There is no history of trauma. On arrival to A&E, he is flushed, dehydrated and pyrexial. All movements of his right hip appear to cause pain. Routine blood tests reveal a WCC of 15.1 × 10^9/l, CRP 234 mg/l and ESR 65 mm/h.

O   153   A 14-year-old boy presents with a limp to the right-hand side. There is no history of trauma. He complains of pain around his right knee, and painful movements of the right knee and hip. He appears small for his age, and has no pubertal hair. On examination he has a full although painful range of movement in his right knee. Movements of the right hip are painful and internal rotation is restricted by 20 degrees.

O   154   An 18-month-old girl with a limp is referred by her general practitioner. She has just started walking. She is otherwise fit and well, and is up to date with all her vaccinations. Perinatal history includes breech delivery and the parents report a club foot which was treated by physiotherapists when she was a neonate.

155 A 4-year-old boy presents with vague pain in the left hip and thigh. Examination reveals a reduced range of internal rotation and abduction. X-rays show flattening and deformity of the femoral head.

THEME: STERILISATION

A   Glutaraldehyde 2%

B   Hot air sterilisation 160 °C for 2 hours

C   Irradiation

D   Steam sterilisation – 15 minutes at 121 °C

E   Steam sterilisation – 15 minutes at 134 °C

For each of the following situations, choose the most appropriate form of sterilisation from the list above. You may use each option once, more than once or not at all.

O   156   Sterilisation of a minor instrument set.

O   157   Sterilisation of a colonoscope.

O   158   Sterilisation of a single-use stapling gun.

THEME: CONSENT

A Accept wishes for non-treatment

B Obtain consent from next of kin

C Proceed to treat without consent of patient

D Section under Mental Health Act to treat

E Seek second opinion

F Requires order from court of law to treat

For each of the following situations, choose the most appropriate option from the list above. Each option may be used once, more than once or not at all.

○ 159 A 43-year-old man with chronic depression attends with sudden-onset abdominal pain. He is peritonitic and has air under his diaphragm. Your consultant has asked you to obtain consent for a laparotomy. The patient refuses and states he would rather die.

○ 160 A 13-year-old has an off-ended distal radial and ulna fracture. On examination she has signs of median nerve compromise. You have spoken with both the girl and her mother and informed them that an operation is necessary. The mother is happy to proceed. The child is adamant that she does not wish to have an operation even though she might not regain full use of her hand.

○ 161 An 84-year-old with known multi-infarct dementia has a fractured neck of femur. He keeps shouting that he wants to be left alone to die.

○ 162 A 64-year-old man is brought into A&E unconscious. He is thought to have a perforated peptic ulcer secondary to NSAID use. He is known to have metastatic carcinoma of the prostate. His wife attends with an advance directive stating that he does not wish any form of surgery or resuscitation.

THEME: UROLOGICAL INVESTIGATIONS

A Abdominal ultrasound

B CT Scan

C Intravenous urography

D Plain radiograph (KUB)

E Radionucleotide imaging

F Transrectal ultrasound

G Uroflowmetry

H Video urodynamics

For each of the following scenarios, choose the most appropriate investigation from the list above. Each option may be used once, more than once or not at all.

163 A 64-year-old man is referred by his general practitioner with a PSA of 11.0 ng/ml. DRE reveals a 50-g craggy-feeling prostate.

164 A 84-year-old man with known metastatic carcinoma of the prostate attends A&E. He is complaining of abdominal pain and has not passed urine in 18 hours. Clinical examination reveals a tender abdomen, with increased tenderness around the renal angles. DRE reveals a 50-g craggy prostate. He is catheterised and has a residual volume of 35 ml.

165 A 46-year-old man presents with a single episode of haematuria. Flexible cystoscopy is performed in clinic, revealing normal-looking bladder and urethral mucosa.

166 A 17-year-old boy presents with a left-sided scrotal swelling. A scrotal ultrasound reveals a varicocele.

ARTERIAL BLOOD GASES

A Compensated metabolic acidosis

B Compensated metabolic alkalosis

C Compensated respiratory acidosis

D Compensated respiratory alkalosis

E Metabolic acidosis

F Metabolic alkalosis

G Respiratory acidosis

H Respiratory alkalosis

For each of the following situations, choose the most appropriate diagnosis from the list above. You may use each option once, more than once or not at all.

167 A 28-year-old woman with acute pancreatitis presents with severe epigastric pain and vomiting. Her blood gases are: pH 7.5; $Pa(O_2)$ 13.9 kPa; $Pa(CO_2)$ 5 kPa; and bicarbonate 33 mmol/l.

168 A 52-year-old diabetic patient attends pre-admission clinic. He appears to be short of breath. His blood gases are: pH 7.31; $Pa(O_2)$ 14.8 kPa; $Pa(CO_2)$ 3 kPa; and bicarbonate 18 mmol/l.

169 A 64-year-old patient in the ICU on her first post-op day following an open aortic aneurysm repair. Her blood gases are: pH 7.31; $Pa(O_2)$ 6.6 kPa; $Pa(CO_2)$ 7.25 kPa; and bicarbonate 24 mmol/l.

THEME: OBSTRUCTIVE JAUNDICE

A Acute pancreatitis

B Biliary colic

C Carcinoma of the pancreas

D Cholangiocarcinoma

E Cholecystitis

F Chronic pancreatitis

G Sclerosing cholangitis

For each of the following scenarios, choose the most likely diagnosis from the list above. Each option may be used once, more than once or not at all.

170 A 72-year-old woman presents with jaundice and RUQ pain. On examination she has a palpable mass in the RUQ. Ultrasound scan of the abdomen reveals dilated ducts, but no gallstones are seen.

171 A 43-year-old presents with a 2-week history of jaundice and steatorrhoea. He has a long-term history of ulcerative colitis, which is treated currently with azathioprine.

172 A 56-year-old alcoholic presents with jaundice and recurrent episodes of severe epigastric pain radiating to the back. Liver function tests show: bilirubin 143 μmol/l, alkaline phosphatase 750 IU/l, aspartate aminotransferase 378 IU/l, gamma-glutaryl transferase 1106 IU/l. Her amylase is 121 IU/l.

173 A 33-year-old woman presents to A&E with severe RUQ pain. The pain has been coming and going for the past 2 hours. Full blood count, urea and electrolytes and liver function test results are all normal. On the consultant ward round the next morning her pain has gone and she wishes to go home.

THEME: STAGING OF TUMOURS

A Ann Arbor staging

B Breslow's staging

C Clark's staging

D Duke's staging

E Gleason's score

F Manchester staging

For each of the following scenarios, choose the most appropriate staging method from the list above. Each option may be used once, more than once or not at all.

○ 174 An excised melanoma found to have a maximum depth of invasion of 6 mm.

○ 175 A 24-year-old presents with a palpable lymph node in the anterior triangle of the neck. Fine-needle aspiration shows the presence of Reed–Sternberg cells.

○ 176 A 73-year-old man presents with PSA of 17.6 ng/ml. A transrectal ultrasound-guided biopsy is performed.

THEME: LOWER LIMB NEUROPATHY

A Common peroneal nerve

B Deep peroneal nerve

C Saphenous nerve

D Sciatic nerve

E Superficial peroneal nerve

F Sural nerve

G Tibial nerve

In the following scenarios which is the most likely nerve to be affected? Each option may be used once, more than once or not at all.

177 A 24-year-old woman was in a below-knee plaster cast for 6 weeks to immobilise a fracture of the distal fibula. On removal of the cast after 6 weeks, she is unable to dorsiflex or evert has no sensation on the dorsum of her foot up to the second interdigital cleft.

178 A 37-year-old woman reattends clinic following treatment of her short saphenous vein varicosities by multiple stab avulsions. She is complaining of numbness along the lateral border of the foot.

179 A 24-year-old man is involved in an RTA. He has a fracture dislocation of the left hip. Following reduction and internal fixation, he is unable to plantar-flex or dorsiflex his foot. He has no sensation below the knee except for the medial aspect of his leg and the upper medial calf.

180 A 69-year-old diabetic man complains of numbness around the medial aspect of the leg following femoro-popliteal bypass grafting using a reversed vein graft.

QUESTIONS
PRACTICE PAPER 3

THEME: OBSTRUCTION

A   Paralytic ileus

B   Adhesions

C   Hernia

D   Volvulus

E   Carcinoma

F   Crohn's disease

G   Gallstone ileus

H   TB

For each of the following scenarios, choose the most likely diagnosis from the list of options above. Each option may be used once, more than once or not at all.

1   A 25-year-old woman with a history of eating disorders and laxative abuse presents with increasing abdominal pain, distension and absolute constipation for 4 days.

2   A 65-year-old man with a 2-month history of altered bowel habit and weight loss presents with a 2-day history of increasing abdominal distension, pain and absolute constipation.

3   A 90-year-old woman 5 days post-op following a hemiarthroplasty of the left hip has increasing abdominal distension and pain and has not opened her bowels for 9 days.

4   A 46-year-old woman who has previously had a hysterectomy and several episodes of abdominal pain presents with increasing pain, distension and absolute constipation. Abdominal X-ray shows distended bowel loops and the biliary tree is outlined.

THEME: INVESTIGATION OF RENAL TRAUMA

A Plain X-ray

B KUB study

C Ultrasound scan (USS)

D IVU

E Cystogram

F Urethrogram

G CT scan

H CT scan with contrast

I Arteriography

For each of the following scenarios, choose the most appropriate investigation from the list above. Each option may be used once, more than once or not at all.

5   An 18-year-old motorcyclist involved in a high-speed RTA sustains multiple injuries, including a head injury, haemothorax, fractured pelvis and femur. There is blood at the external urethral meatus.

6   A 45-year-old man involved in an RTA as the restrained driver sustains fractures of ribs 8–12. He is initially haemodynamically unstable, but responds to fluids. There is free fluid in the abdomen on a FAST scan (focused abdominal sonography for trauma) and frank haematuria is draining from the catheter.

7   A 25-year-old man sustains a stab wound to the left flank. He has haematuria draining from his catheter and severe left loin pain.

8   A 30-year-old motorcyclist sustains an unstable pelvic fracture. His catheter is draining frank haematuria.

THEME: BURNS

A 1%

B 1.25%

C 2.5%

D 9%

E 10%

F 18%

G 19%

H 27%

I 36%

J 45%

For each of the following scenarios, choose the correct percentage surface area of burn from the list above. Each option may be used once, more than once or not at all.

○ 9 A 37-year-old man is brought into A&E with red, blistered burns affecting the anterior aspects of both legs and the perineum.

○ 10 An 18-year-old woman presents to A&E having picked up a hot pan. She has red, painful, blistered burns on the palms of both hands.

○ 11 A 69-year-old man is brought to A&E following a house fire, with black, insensate burns covering the trunk and red, painful burns to the anterior and posterior aspects of the right arm.

○ 12 A 45-year-old woman presents to A&E with painful, red, blistered burns covering the head and neck, and pink, unblistered skin on the right palm.

THEME: STATISTICS

A Quantitative measured data

B Quantitative counted data

C Ordinal data

D Nominal data

For each of the following, choose the most appropriate option from the list above. Each option may be used once, more than once or not at all.

○   13   Blood groups.

○   14   Blood pressure.

○   15   Staging of colorectal cancer.

THEME: DRAINS

A Closed non-suction drain

B Closed suction drain

C Corrugated drain

D No drain required

E Sump drain

F T-tube

For each of the following situations, choose the most appropriate drain from the list above. Each option may be used once, more than once or not at all.

○ 16 Bowel anastomosis following uncomplicated elective surgery.

○ 17 Immediately following thyroidectomy.

○ 18 A high-output enteric fistula.

○ 19 A skin flap.

○ 20 An oesophageal perforation.

PAPER 3 QUESTIONS

THEME: FRACTURE CLASSIFICATIONS

A Colton's classification

B Garden's classification

C Gustilo–Anderson classification

D Mason's classification

E Neer's classification

F Salter–Harris classification

G Weber's classification

For each of the following scenarios, choose the most appropriate option from the list above. Each option may be used once, more than once or not at all.

○ 21 An open tibial fracture.

○ 22 A displaced radial head fracture.

○ 23 A fractured distal radius in an 11-year-old child.

○ 24 An intracapsular fractured neck of femur.

THEME: LOCAL ANAESTHETICS

A Bupivacaine

B Bupivacaine and adrenaline

C Bupivacaine and lidocaine

D Lidocaine

E Lidocaine and adrenaline

F Prilocaine

G Ropivacaine

For each of the following situations, choose the most appropriate option from the list above. Each option may be used once, more than once or not at all.

25 For a digital nerve block to allow suturing of a clean laceration.

26 For Bier's block to manipulate a Colles' fracture.

27 Excision of a sebaceous cyst from the scalp.

28 For post-operative analgesia after Zadik's procedure under a general anaesthetic.

29 For a spinal anaesthetic.

THEME: TREATMENT OF FRACTURES

A Broad arm sling

B Intramedullary nail

C Manipulation under anaesthetic

D Open reduction and internal fixation

E Thomas' splint

F Traction

For each of the following situations, choose the most appropriate treatment option from the list above. Each option may be used once, more than once or not at all.

O   30   A closed fracture of the lateral malleolus above the level of the syndesmosis with talar shift.

O   31   An undisplaced fracture of the radial head in the patient's non-dominant arm.

O   32   A closed femoral shaft fracture in a patient injured in an RTA who has also sustained fractures of the tibia and fibula on the same side, and radius and ulna on the opposite side.

O   33   An undisplaced clavicle fracture, with no compromise of the overlying skin.

THEME: THE LIMPING CHILD

A Osteomyelitis

B Perthes' disease

C Septic arthritis

D SUFE

E Transient synovitis

F Tubercular arthritis

For each of the following scenarios, choose the most appropriate option from the list above. Each option may be used once, more than once or not at all.

34 A 6-year-old boy, weighing 15 kg, presents with a few days history of limp. He complains of intermittent right hip and thigh pain, of which he has previously had less severe episodes.

35 A 6-year-old boy presents with a 2-day history of left hip and thigh pain. He had a recent sore throat which has now resolved. He is apyrexial. On examination internal rotation is decreased. His WCC is 7×10^9/l, erythrocyte sedimentation rate (ESR) is 2 mm/h and C-reactive protein (CRP) is 2 mg/l.

36 A 2-year-old boy with a chest infection is pyrexial and cries on all movements of the right leg.

37 A 14-year-old boy, weighing 70 kg, presents with pain in the right thigh and knee and a decreased range of abduction.

THEME: FRACTURED NECK OF FEMUR

A Austin Moore hemiarthroplasty

B Closed reduction and cannulated screws

C Dynamic hip screw

D Immediate cannulated screws

E Thompson's hemiarthroplasty

F Total hip replacement

G Open reduction and internal fixation

For each of the following scenarios, choose the most appropriate treatment option from the list above. Each option may be used once, more than once or not at all.

○ 38 A 75-year-old woman tripped on the pavement and has a displaced subcapital fractured left neck of femur. Her only past medical history is hypertension.

○ 39 A previously fit and well 60-year-old woman fell downstairs, sustaining a minimally displaced subcapital fracture of the left neck of femur.

○ 40 An 82-year-old with a previous history of myocardial infarction fell while walking the dog. He sustains a two-part inter-trochanteric fracture of the right neck of femur.

○ 41 A 26-year-old man is involved in an RTA and injures his right hip. An X-ray shows a displaced (Garden III) subcapital fractured neck of femur.

○ 42 A 77-year-old woman trips while shopping, sustaining an inter-trochanteric fracture of the left neck of femur. There is a 6-cm subtrochanteric extension.

THEME: ISCHAEMIC LIMBS

A Amputation

B Angiogram

C Angiogram and bypass

D Angiogram and thrombolysis

E Angioplasty

F Best medical therapy

G Embolectomy

H Intravenous heparin

I Reconstruction

For each of the following scenarios, choose the most appropriate option from the list above. Each option may be used once, more than once or not at all.

43 A patient presents with a history of sudden onset of a painful, cold, numb left foot. There are no previous symptoms. The pulse is irregularly irregular, with no pulses below the femoral in the left leg and all pulses present in right leg.

44 A patient with congestive cardiac failure (CCF) who is on a medical ward develops a sudden-onset cold, pulseless, numb right foot. Dorsalis pedis and posterior tibial pulses are absent on the right and all pulses are present on left.

45 A diabetic patient who has been on the ward for several weeks for treatment of large infected foot ulcers develops three black toes on the right foot.

46 A 64-year-old man, a heavy smoker, has a history of intermittent claudication affecting the right calf. He presents with an acutely ischaemic right leg. On examination the limb is found to have lost sensation. Angiography shows occlusion of the right femoral artery with good distal run-off,

THEME: ABDOMINAL AORTIC ANEURYSMS

A CT scan

B Emergency surgery

C Elective endoluminal repair

D Elective open repair

E Urgent elective repair

F Ultrasound in 6 months

G Ultrasound in 1 year

For each of the following scenarios, choose the most appropriate option from the list above. Each option may be used once, more than once or not at all.

47 A patient seen in clinic following an asymptomatic 3.5-cm AAA being discovered during an ultrasound of the renal tract.

48 A patient known to have an AAA, which was 5.3 cm at the previous clinic appointment, has undergone a CT scan. The scan reveals a 5.7-cm infrarenal aneurysm extending from 0.5 cm below the renal arteries into both common iliacs.

49 A patient known to have an AAA is reviewed in clinic for the third time. Ultrasound reveals an increase in size from 4 cm to 4.5 cm.

50 An asymptomatic patient is reviewed in clinic. The ultrasound shows a 5-cm AAA. A scan taken 6 months before showed a 3.7-cm aneurysm.

THEME: CAROTID ARTERY DISEASE

A Best medical therapy

B Endarterectomy left side

C Endarterectomy right side

For each of the following scenarios, choose the most appropriate option from the list above. Each option may be used once, more than once or not at all.

51 A fit and well 76-year-old patient presents with a history of right-sided facial drooping lasting approximately 12 hours, then fully resolving. Duplex scans show a bilateral carotid artery stenosis of 86%.

52 A 73-year-old woman presents with three episodes of amaurosis fugax affecting the right eye during the past 6 months. Duplex scans reveal a bilateral stenosis of 75%.

53 An 87-year-old man presents with an episode of right-sided hemiparesis which fully resolves after 1 week. Duplex scans show a right-sided stenosis of 100% and a left-sided stenosis of 50%.

54 An 82-year-old woman presents with a history of one episode of vertigo and diplopia resolving within 24 hours. Duplex scans show a left-sided stenosis of 60%.

THEME: HEAD INJURIES

A Admission for neurological observations

B CT scan

C Home with advice

D Intubation and ventilation

E Referral to neurosurgery

F Skull X-ray

For each of the following scenarios, choose the most appropriate option from the list above. Each option may be used once, more than once or not at all.

55 A 50-year-old man falls and bangs his head on a cupboard. He cannot remember the events of the fall, but remembers everything since. He had a loss of consciousness of approximately 30 seconds witnessed by his wife, who lives with him.

56 A 70-year-old man on warfarin for atrial fibrillation trips and falls. There is no loss of consciousness, but he has large laceration over the occiput. He lives with his wife.

57 A 30-year-old woman is hit with a metal bar. She has a depressed skull fracture on X-ray. Her Glasgow Coma Scale (GCS) score is 15.

58 A 35-year-old woman has a head injury in an RTA. She remembers the events and did not lose consciousness. Her GCS is 15 throughout. She has a left haemotympanum on examination.

THEME: BLOOD GAS ANALYSIS

A Respiratory alkalosis

B Respiratory acidosis with compensation

C Respiratory acidosis without compensation

D Metabolic alkalosis

E Metabolic acidosis with compensation

F Metabolic acidosis without compensation

For each of the following situations, choose the most appropriate diagnosis from the list above. You may use each option once, more than once or not at all.

O 59 pH 7.47; Pa(O_2) 12.3 kPa; Pa(CO_2) 4.8 kPa; bicarbonate 25 mmol/l; base excess +5 mmol/l.

O 60 pH 7.31; Pa(O_2) 12.7 kPa; Pa(CO_2) 3.2 kPa; bicarbonate 19 mmol/l; base excess −7 mmol/l.

O 61 pH 7.29; Pa(O_2) 8.4 kPa; Pa(CO_2) 6.7 kPa; bicarbonate 32 mmol/l; base excess −1 mmol/l.

O 62 pH 7.28; Pa(O_2) 13.8 kPa; Pa(CO_2) 5.0 kPa; bicarbonate 20 mmol/l; base excess −8 mmol/l.

THEME: CONSENT

A Doctor can consent for the patient

B Patient can give valid consent

C Patient's refusal is valid and doctor cannot override

D Parents can consent for the patient

E Refusal is not valid and can be overridden

For each of the following situations, choose the most appropriate option from the list above. Each option may be used once, more than once or not at all.

63 A 24-year-old nurse presents with testicular torsion. He refuses surgery despite having had the benefits and risks of the procedure explained.

64 A 15-year-old girl whose parents are abroad requires an emergency appendicectomy. She understands the operation, its benefits and risks.

65 An 86-year-old woman with dementia, mini-mental state score 4/10, is admitted with a fractured neck of femur. Her daughter states that she would not have wanted surgery, but there is no advance directive.

66 A 15-year-old boy needs an appendicectomy. His parents refuse the surgery despite hearing the risks and benefits, but the patient gives consent. The patient has five GCSEs.

THEME: SCROTAL SWELLINGS

A Epididymal cyst

B Epididymo-orchitis

C Gumma

D Hernia

E Hydrocoele

F Spermatocele

G Testicular torsion

H Testicular tumour

I Varicocele

For each of the following scenarios, choose the most appropriate option from the list above. Each option may be used once, more than once or not at all.

○ 67 The patient has a right-sided swelling in the scrotum separate from the testis, which you cannot get above. The swelling transmits a cough impulse.

○ 68 The patient has a left-sided swelling and dull ache for 1–2 weeks. The swelling is separate from the testis and transilluminates.

○ 69 The patient has a generalised, non-tender swelling of the left hemiscrotum, which has been gradually increasing in size for 2 months. The testis and epididymis cannot be defined. The swelling transilluminates.

○ 70 A 28-year-old man presents with a 6-hour history of a painful right hemiscrotum. The testis and epididymis can be defined, with a normal lie of the testis, and the epididymis is tender to palpation. The patient has been feeling generally unwell and has had dysuria for 2 days.

71   A 20-year-old man presents with a 2-hour history of severe right-sided testicular pain and swelling. The hemiscrotum is very tender, with the testis lying normally.

THEME: TUMOUR MARKERS

A Adrenocorticotropic hormone (ACTH)

B CA 19-9

C CA 125

D Calcitonin

E Carcinoembryonic antigen (CEA)

F α-Fetoprotein

G γ-Glutamyl transferase (GGT)

H β-Human chorionic gonadotropin (hCG)

I Lactate dehydrogenase

J Prostate-specific antigen (PSA)

For each of the following malignancies, choose the most appropriate marker from the list above. Each option may be used once, more than once or not at all.

◯ 72 Colorectal carcinoma.

◯ 73 Breast cancer.

◯ 74 Ovarian cancer.

◯ 75 Prostate cancer.

◯ 76 Choriocarcinoma.

◯ 77 Small-cell lung cancer.

THEME: CONGENITAL GASTROINTESTINAL ANOMALIES

A Duodenal atresia

B Exomphalos

C Gastroschisis

D Hirschsprung's disease

E Hypertrophic pyloric stenosis

F Meconium ileus

G Oesophageal atresia

H Small-bowel atresia

For each of the following scenarios, choose the most likely anomaly from the list above. Each option may be used once, more than once or not at all.

78 Neonate girl, born at term, presents with uncovered intestine and an ovary protruding through the abdominal wall to the right of the umbilicus, through a defect of approximately 3 cm.

79 A term neonate boy, who has failed to pass meconium, has now developed bilious vomiting and abdominal distension. Per rectal examination reveals a mucus plug, removal of which temporarily relieves the symptoms, but they recur.

80 A neonate girl presents with bilious vomiting and abdominal distension. She passed meconium, but has not opened her bowels since. An abdominal X-ray reveals distended bowel loops with fluid levels.

81 A neonate boy with trisomy 21 presents with bilious vomiting and abdominal distension on day 2. An abdominal X-ray reveals a double gas bubble.

82 A 1-month-old baby boy presents with repeated projectile vomiting of unaltered feed approximately 10 minutes after feeding.

THEME: TREATMENT OF GALLSTONES

A Elective laparoscopic cholecystectomy

B Elective open cholecystectomy

C Endoscopic retrograde cholangiopancreatography (ERCP) + sphincterotomy

D Low-fat diet

E Urgent cholecystectomy

For each of the following scenarios, choose the most appropriate treatment option from the list above. Each option may be used once, more than once or not at all.

83 A 46-year-old woman with renal calculi has a routine ultrasound which reveals three small stones in the gallbladder.

84 A patient admitted 3 days ago with RUQ pain, vomiting, rigors and a temperature greater than 38 °C, which have failed to settle despite intravenous antibiotics.

85 A 50-year-old man known to have gallstones in the gallbladder, who has had two previous attacks of biliary colic, one requiring hospital admission. He has a past medical history of epilepsy, and a vagotomy and pyloroplasty.

THEME: CHEST INJURIES

A Aortic dissection/disruption

B Cardiac tamponade

C Diaphragmatic rupture

D Flail chest

E Haemothorax

F Oesophageal injury

G Simple pneumothorax

H Tension pneumothorax

I Tracheobronchial injury

For each of the following scenarios, choose the most appropriate option from the list above. Each option may be used once, more than once or not at all.

86 A restrained driver involved in an RTA develops dyspnoea and tachypnoea prior to arrival in A&E. On examination air entry is decreased on the left side of the chest and decreased bowel sounds are audible.

87 A restrained passenger involved in an RTA develops dyspnoea, tachypnoea and tachycardia. On examination chest wall movements are paradoxical.

88 A restrained front-seat passenger involved in an RTA in which a car travelling at high speed collided with a wall was haemodynamically unstable at the scene. Both radial pulses were absent and he went into cardiac arrest at the scene.

89 A restrained back-seat passenger involved in an RTA has remained haemodynamically stable, but is tachypnoeic and dyspnoeic. Examination reveals no tracheal deviation, with decreased chest wall expansion, decreased air entry on the left and a dullness to percussion on this side.

90 A restrained driver involved in a high-speed impact with a tree has stridor, tachypnoea, dyspnoea and subcutaneous emphysema.

91 A 21-year-old is brought to A&E unconscious. He has been involved in an RTA. Primary survey reveals that he is hypotensive and tachycardic, and a chest X-ray reveals a flail chest but no obvious pneumothorax. He has refractory hypotension, with no obvious point of blood loss, so a laparotomy is organised. He is intubated in the department and has a 4-unit blood transfusion started in the department. As he is being transferred to the operating theatre he goes into cardiac arrest.

92 A 29-year-old has a stab injury to the left side of the chest. Primary survey shows a large left haemothorax which is subsequently drained with a water seal chest drain. After 30 minutes he appears to be in significant distress. On examination he is tachycardic at 120 beats/min and his BP is 90/50 mmHg. He appears to have engorgement of his neck veins and his heart sounds are difficult to hear.

93 A 34-year-old is brought in with a stab wound to the right side of his chest. Primary survey shows a tension pneumothorax. This is initially treated with needle thoracocentesis. A chest drain is inserted. A check X-ray 30 minutes after tube insertion shows the tube to be in a satisfactory position. The patient continues to be in respiratory distress and a repeat chest X-ray after 30 minutes shows a persistent large pneumothorax.

THEME: STERILISATION

A Autoclave

B Dry heat

C Ethylene oxide

D Glutaraldehyde

E Irradiation

F Low-temperature steam and formaldehyde

For each of the following, choose the most appropriate form of sterilisation from the list above. You may use each option once, more than once or not at all.

○   94   Catheters.

○   95   Flexible naso-endoscope.

○   96   Sutures.

○   97   Small McIndoe scissors.

THEME: TOURNIQUETS

A No tourniquet

B Simple tourniquet

C Tourniquet at 150 mmHg

D Tourniquet at 200 mmHg

E Tourniquet at 250 mmHg

F Tourniquet at 300 mmHg

For each of the following scenarios, choose the most appropriate tourniquet from the list above. Each option may be used once, more than once or not at all.

○ 98 A patient with a blood pressure of 150/90 mmHg undergoing Zadik's procedure.

○ 99 A patient with a blood pressure of 140/80 mmHg undergoing fasciectomy for Dupuytren's contracture.

○ 100 A patient with a blood pressure of 150/114 mmHg undergoing knee arthroscopy, who has previously had a femoro-popliteal bypass.

THEME: BIOPSY TECHNIQUES

A Brush cytology

B Core biopsy

C Endoscopic biopsy

D Excisional biopsy

E Fine-needle aspiration cytology

F Frozen section

G Incisional biopsy

For each of the following lesions, choose the most appropriate biopsy technique from the list above. Each option may be used once, more than once or not at all.

○   101 A lymph node found during Whipple's procedure.

○   102 A solitary nodule within the thyroid.

○   103 A suspected basal cell carcinoma.

○   104 A mass on the bladder wall.

THEME: PAROTID SWELLINGS

A Acute bacterial sialolithiasis

B Adenocarcinoma

C Adenolymphoma

D Pleomorphic adenoma

E Sarcoidosis

F Sialolithiasis

G Sjögren syndrome

H Squamous cell carcinoma

I Acute viral sialadenitis

J Frey syndrome

K Mikulicz syndrome

For each of the following scenarios, choose the most appropriate diagnosis from the list above. Each option may be used once, more than once or not at all.

○ 105 A 47-year-old man presents with a 6-month history of a slowly growing, smooth lesion in the right parotid. All facial movements are normal.

○ 106 A 70-year-old man presents with a painless swelling of the left parotid which he has had for 3 months. He previously had surgery for a right parotid lesion. All facial movements are normal.

○ 107 A 70-year-old man presents with a rapidly growing, painful, hard, left parotid lump, which has been there for 1 month. The left side of his mouth is drooping. He has previously had radiotherapy to his parathyroids.

○ 108 A 64-year-old man attends for routine post-operative follow-up following surgery to remove a stone from his parotid gland. He now complains of diffuse facial sweating before meals.

109 A 21-year-old man presents with bilateral tender swellings of his parotid glands along with bilaterally tender testes.

110 A 43-year-old woman with a history of systemic lupus erythematosus (SLE) presents with a severe dry mouth and dry eyes.

111 A 79-year-old woman with recently diagnosed acute lymphocytic leukaemia presents with symmetrical enlargement of all salivary glands, narrowing of her palpebral fissures and a dry mouth.

112 A 59-year-old woman presents with left parotid swelling. It occurs immediately before meals and is exquisitely tender.

THEME: JOINT INFECTIONS

A Group B streptococcus

B Haemolytic streptococcus

C *Haemophilus influenzae*

D *Neisseria gonorrhoeae*

E *Staphylococcus aureus*

For each of the following situations, choose the most appropriate organism from the list above. Each option may be used once, more than once or not at all.

○ 113 Septic arthritis in a 2-year-old child.

○ 114 Septic arthritis in a 9-year-old child.

○ 115 Osteomyelitis in a 49-year-old man.

THEME: SUTURE MATERIALS

A 1 PDS (polydioxanone suture)

B 3-0 PDS

C 3-0 Prolene

D 6-0 Prolene

E 3-0 Nylon

F Steel wire

G 3-0 Vicryl

H 1 Vicryl

For each of the following situations, choose the most appropriate suture material from the list above. Each option may be used once, more than once or not at all.

○ 116 Distal sutures for a femoro-distal anastomosis.

○ 117 Abdominal mass closure following laparotomy.

○ 118 Interrupted sutures following Dupuytren's contracture surgery.

○ 119 Sternal closure following bypass surgery.

○ 120 An absorbable suture commonly used for bowel anastomosis.

THEME: MULTIPLE ENDOCRINE NEOPLASIA

A Gorlin syndrome

B Sipple syndrome

C Werner syndrome

For each of the following descriptions, choose the most appropriate MEN syndrome from the list above. Each option may be used once, more than once or not at all.

○ 121 A very tall 20-year-old man with a high, arched palate, large span and long fingers, presenting with a medullary thyroid carcinoma.

○ 122 A 40-year-old woman presents with bilateral phaeochromocytoma. She has a past medical history of medullary thyroid carcinoma.

○ 123 A 50-year-old woman presents with pituitary adenoma and parathyroid hyperplasia. Her mother also had a pituitary adenoma.

○ 124 A 60-year-old man who has multiple mucosal neuromas presents with a medullary thyroid carcinoma.

THEME: TYPES OF GRAFT

A Allogenic heterotropic graft

B Allogenic orthotopic graft

C Autogenic graft

D Xenogenic heterotropic graft

E Xenogenic orthotopic graft

For each of the following situations, choose the most appropriate description from the list above. Each option may be used once, more than once or not at all.

O   125 A kidney transplant from mother to son.

O   126 A baboon's heart into a human recipient.

O   127 A full-thickness skin graft.

O   128 Pancreas from an unrelated human donor to a recipient.

THEME: UPPER GASTROINTESTINAL HAEMORRHAGE

A Aorto-enteric fistula

B Duodenal ulcer

C Gastric malignancy

D Gastric ulcer

E Mallory–Weiss tear

F Oesophageal varices

G Oesophagitis

H Vascular malformation

For each of the following scenarios, choose the most appropriate diagnosis from the list above. Each option may be used once, more than once or not at all.

129 A 80-year-old woman presents with haematemesis. She has had intermittent epigastric pain after food for the past 6 months. She has lost weight – about 3.5 kg (half a stone). She was recently commenced on diclofenac.

130 A 21-year-old student presents with haematemesis. He drank a large amount of alcohol last night and was retching prior to the haematemesis.

131 A 50-year-old man presents with a massive haematemesis. He is haemodynamically unstable. He has clubbing, palmar erythema, gynaecomastia and hepatomegaly.

132 A 30-year-old man presents with haematemesis. He complains of a year-long history of epigastric pain relieved by eating. He is a smoker.

133 A 64-year-old man presents with haematemesis and melaena. He is haemodynamically unstable. He has a previous history of an AAA repair 15 years ago.

THEME: LOWER GASTROINTESTINAL HAEMORRHAGE

A Angiodysplasia

B Colorectal cancer

C Crohn's disease

D Diverticular disease

E Haemorrhoids

F Infection

G Ulcerative colitis

For each of the following scenarios, choose the most appropriate option from the list above. Each option may be used once, more than once or not at all.

134 A 40-year-old patient presents with recurrent episodes of fresh bleeding per rectum, with no associated abdominal pain. Fresh blood, but no mass is found on rectal examination. The patient has telangiectasia on the face and mouth. His haemoglobin is 9.2 g/dl.

135 A 25-year-old woman presents with a 1-month history of worsening intermittent bloody diarrhoea with mucus, associated with crampy abdominal pain. She has lost 3.5 kg (half a stone). There is clubbing of her fingers.

136 A 70-year-old woman presents with a large, fresh rectal bleed. She has no abdominal pain. She gives a history of altered bowel habit and left-sided abdominal pain relieved by defecation for 1 year. She has not lost any weight.

137 A 75-year-old man presents with a painless rectal bleed. He complains of altered bowel habit and tenesmus for a month, associated with smaller rectal bleeds. He has lost 1.5 kg (quarter of a stone).

138 A 30-year-old pregnant woman presents with fresh bleeding per rectum, which she has noticed on the toilet paper.

THEME: FLUIDS

A 0 mmol/l

B 4 mmol/l

C 4.5 mmol/l

D 5 mmol/l

E 30 mmol/l

F 50 mmol/l

G 130 mmol/l

H 142 mmol/l

I 154 mmol/l

For each of the following statements, choose the most appropriate concentration from the list above. Each option may be used once, more than once or not at all.

○ 139 The sodium concentration of serum.

○ 140 The sodium concentration of Hartmann's solution.

○ 141 The sodium concentration of Gelofusine.

○ 142 The sodium concentration of 4% dextrose saline.

○ 143 The potassium concentration of Gelofusine.

THEME: NUTRITIONAL SUPPORT

A Jejunostomy

B Nasogastric feeding

C Nasojejunal feeding

D Oral supplementation

E Percutaneous endoscopic gastrostomy (PEG) feeding

F Total parenteral nutrition (TPN)

For each of the following patients, choose the most appropriate form of nutritional support from the list above. Each option may be used once, more than once or not at all.

○ 147 A patient with severe acute pancreatitis.

○ 148 A patient who has had a CVA affecting their swallowing a week ago.

○ 149 A patient undergoing Whipple's procedure.

○ 150 A patient with Crohn's disease affecting the small bowel.

THEME: HYPOVOLAEMIC SHOCK

A   Class I hypovolaemic shock

B   Class II hypovolaemic shock

C   Class III hypovolaemic shock

D   Class IV hypovolaemic shock

**For each of the following scenarios, choose the most appropriate op
from the list above. Each option may be used once, more than once
not at all.**

O   144   An 18-year-old man involved in an RTA has a fractured right
femur and open fracture of the left tibia. His pulse is 109/min
regular, BP 114/90 mmHg and RR 25 breaths/min.

O   145   A 50-year-old man with a bleeding peptic ulcer. His pulse is
98/min, BP 134/72 mmHg and RR 20 breaths/min.

O   146   A 30-year-old pregnant woman with a per vaginal bleed. Her
pulse is 138/min, BP 92/70 mmHg, RR 35 breaths/min.

THEME: THYROID NEOPLASMS

A Anaplastic carcinoma

B Follicular carcinoma

C Malignant lymphoma

D Medullary carcinoma

E Metastases

F Papillary carcinoma

For each of the following scenarios, choose the most appropriate malignancy from the list above. Each option may be used once, more than once or not at all.

151 A 35-year-old woman presents with a painless nodule, gradually increasing in size, in the left lobe of the thyroid. Histological examination reveals psammoma bodies.

152 An 83-year-old woman presents with a rapidly growing hard painless lump in the right lobe of the thyroid, associated with dysphagia.

153 A 47-year-old woman presents with a painless lump, gradually increasing in size, in the left lobe of the thyroid. Her serum calcitonin level is elevated.

THEME: NIPPLE DISCHARGE

A Ductal carcinoma in situ

B Duct ectasia

C Intraductal papilloma

D Periductal mastitis

E Physiological discharge

F Prolactinoma

For each of the following scenarios, choose the most appropriate diagnosis from the list above. Each option may be used once, more than once or not at all.

O 154 A 20-year-old woman with a bloody single-duct discharge and a palpable mass at the areola. No malignant cells are isolated from the discharge.

O 155 A 31-year-old woman, a smoker, with a purulent discharge associated with tenderness.

O 156 A 62-year-old woman with a bloody single-duct discharge. There is no palpable mass.

O 157 A 33-year-old multiparous woman presents with a multiductal white discharge, no blood on dipstick. She is being investigated for weight gain and irregular menstruation.

THEME: SHOULDER PAIN

A Acute calcific tendonitis

B Acute dislocation

C Frozen shoulder

D Glenohumeral arthritis

E Recurrent dislocation

F Referred from cervical spine

G Rotator cuff tear

H Subacromial impingement

PAPER 3 QUESTIONS

For each of the following scenarios, choose the most appropriate option from the list above. Each option may be used once, more than once or not at all.

158 A 25-year-old woman presents with a 12-hour history of rapidly increasing severe right shoulder pain, worst on abduction between 120 and 170 degrees.

159 An 18-year-old rugby player presents with severe left shoulder pain following a direct blow to the shoulder. The left shoulder appears flattened.

160 A 73-year-old man presents 3 days after a fall with a painful left shoulder. The pain is worse at night and he is unable to lie on that side. Abduction and external rotation are severely decreased, and all movements are painful.

THEME: ASA GRADING – CLASSIFICATION OF PHYSICAL STATUS

A Class 1

B Class 2

C Class 3

D Class 4

E Class 5

For each of the following patients select the most appropriate ASA (American Society of Anesthesiologists) grade. Each option may be used once, more than once or not at all.

○ 161 A 54-year-old man with chronic renal failure, requiring dialysis. He wants to have a total hip replacement for severe osteoarthritis.

○ 162 A 64-year-old woman with tablet-controlled hypertension for whom a laparoscopic cholecystectomy has been planned.

○ 163 A 34-year-old man ruptures his anterior cruciate ligament (ACL) playing football and needs to have it repaired.

○ 164 A 32-year-old patient with a 10-year history of ulcerative colitis, fully controlled with medication, due to undergo varicose vein stripping in the lower limbs.

○ 165 An 18-year-old man due to undergo inguinal hernia repair. He has a history of severe asthma that needed ICU admission in the past. He has to use inhalers four times a day, and is admitted to hospital with an acute exacerbation at least twice a year.

THEME: STAGING OF TRANSITIONAL CELL CARCINOMA OF BLADDER

A T_{is}

B T_1

C T_{2a}

D T_{2b}

E T_{3a}

F T_{3b}

G T_{4a}

H T_{4b}

For each of the following scenarios, choose the most appropriate option from the list above. Each option may be used once, more than once or not at all.

○ 166 A 67-year-old woman presents with a several-month history of painless haematuria. Ultrasound of the upper tracts in normal but urine cytological examination is positive for malignant cells. Bimanual examination under general anaesthetic shows that the tumour is fixed to the left lateral side wall.

○ 167 A 70-year-old man presents for 6-monthly surveillance cystoscopy following a diagnosis and resection of transitional cell carcinoma bladder (stage T_1) 2 years ago. A suspicious area is seen and TURBT is carried out. Histological examination shows that the tumour breaches the lamina propria and invades the superficial muscle.

THEME: POLYPS

A Fibroma

B Hyperplastic polyp

C Inflammatory polyp

D Juvenile polyp

E Peutz–Jeghers polyp

F Tubular adenoma

G Villous adenoma

For each of the descriptions below, select the most likely type of polyp. Each option may be used once, more than once or not at all.

○ 168 The most common polyp found in children. Present as PR bleeding or by prolapsing through the anus. Not pre-malignant.

○ 169 Rare colonic tumour which arises from the submucosal layer. Can contain muscle or glandular tissue.

○ 170 Most common type of polyp, usually found in the rectum. No evidence that they undergo malignant change.

THEME: RADIOLOGICAL APPEARANCES

A Diverticular disease

B Duodenal atresia

C Hirschprung's disease

D Necrotising enterocolitis

E Perforated duodenal ulcer

F Sigmoid volvulus

G Ulcerative colitis

For each of the X-ray descriptions below, select the most likely diagnosis from the list above. Each option may be used once, more than once or not at all.

171 Distended loop of bowel and 'beak sign' on instant enema.

172 Tubular shaped colon with no faecal matter within the affected part of the bowel.

THEME: PERIPHERAL NERVE INJURY

A Axillary nerve

B Median nerve

C Musculocutaneous nerve

D Posterior interosseous nerve of the forearm

E Radial nerve

F Ulnar nerve

In the following scenarios, which is the most likely nerve to be affected? Each option may be used once, more than once or not at all.

○ 173 A 21-year-old man suffers an anterior dislocation of his right shoulder. Examination after reduction reveals an area of sensory loss around the lateral aspect of the shoulder.

○ 174 A 53-year-old woman falls onto an outstretched hand. X-rays of the elbow reveal a fracture of the radial neck. She has no sensory loss, but has weak extension of the wrist and cannot extend her fingers.

○ 175 A 66-year-old woman falls, fracturing the surgical neck of humerus. Six months after the injury she continues to struggle to abduct her shoulder.

○ 176 An 8-year-old boy has a supracondylar fracture of the right elbow. After initial K-wire fixation he reattends the clinic for routine follow-up. There is hyperextension of the metacarpophalangeal joints of the ring and little fingers and flexion of the interphalangeal joints.

○ 177 A 23-year-old man has a deep laceration to the anterior aspect of his arm. When seen in A&E there is pulsatile bleeding from the wound and he is unable to flex at the wrist.

ANSWERS

ANSWERS
PRACTICE PAPER 1

DIATHERMY

1   A – Monopolar diathermy

2   B – Bipolar diathermy

3   D – Coagulation

4   B – Bipolar diathermy

5   A – Monopolar diathermy

Monopolar diathermy works with a high-power unit (400 W), passing the current from the active electrode through the patient to the patient plate electrode and back to the generator. It can be used for cutting and buzzing.

Bipolar diathermy works with a low-power unit (50 W), passing the current between the tips of the forceps. It is therefore safer for use in patients with pacemakers and on end-arteries in the extremities, eg digits, scrotum, penis. It cannot be used for cutting or buzzing.

Cutting diathermy works with a continuous output, coagulation with a pulsed, short, high-frequency output, and blend with a combination of the two.

EXTENSOR COMPARTMENTS OF THE WRIST

6   B – II

7   B – II

8   E – V

Table 1   The extensor compartments of the wrist and their contents

Compartment	Contents
I	Abductor pollicis longus Extensor pollicis brevis
II	Extensor carpi radialis brevis Extensor carpi radialis longus
III	Extensor pollicis longus
IV	Extensor indicis Extensor digitorum
V	Extensor digiti minimi
VI	Extensor carpi ulnaris

At the wrist extensor compartment II lies radial to Lister's tubercle and compartment III ulnar to it.

SEPSIS

9   E – Septic shock

10   C – Sepsis

11   A – Bacteraemia

12   B – SIRS

The important definitions concerning sepsis are:

Bacteraemia – the presence of bacteria in the bloodstream.

SIRS – a systemic inflammatory response to a range of insults, with two or more of:

- Temperature $> 38\,°C$ or $< 36\,°C$
- Pulse $< 90/min$
- RR > 20 breaths/min or $Pa(co_2) > 4.3$ kPa
- WCC $> 12 \times 10^9/l$ or $< 4 \times 10^9/l$

Sepsis – SIRS with a documented infection.

Severe sepsis – SIRS with a documented infection and hypotension, hypoperfusion and organ dysfunction.

Septic shock – sepsis with hypotension persisting despite adequate fluid resuscitation.

FACIAL NERVE PALSIES

13   G – Temporal bone fracture

The recent head injury suggests temporal bone fracture, and Battle's sign and haemotympanum are both signs of this.

14   A – Multiple sclerosis

The sparing of the forehead suggests that the cause of the facial nerve palsy is supranuclear. Optic neuritis is a common presentation of multiple sclerosis.

15   H – Ramsay Hunt syndrome

Ramsay Hunt syndrome is herpes zoster. The history of severe pain prior to the palsy and associated vertigo and hearing loss, coupled with papules (which can be present in the ear canal or on the tongue), point to this diagnosis.

16   D – Choleasteatoma

The 2-month history of intermittent discharge is a concerning feature with the facial nerve palsy. Cholesteatomas should not be missed as a diagnosis, and typically cause retraction pockets in the tympanic membrane.

17   B – Acoustic neuroma

The accompanying symptoms, particularly the sensorineural hearing loss, are typical of acoustic neuroma.

18   I – Chronic suppurative otitis media

The history of hearing loss, which is found to be conductive, coupled with a dull tympanic membrane due to fluid collecting behind it, point to chronic suppurative otits media.

ANAESTHETIC AGENTS

19 I – Isoflurane

20 D – Suxamethonium

21 K – Nitrous oxide

22 B – Propofol

Induction agents include:
- Thiopentone sodium
- Propofol
- Etomidate

Propofol is the only one with a slight anti-emetic effect, and is the choice of agent with laryngeal masks.

Depolarising muscle relaxants:
- Suxamethonium

Non-depolarising muscle relaxants:
- Atracurium
- Vercuronium

Inhalational agents include:
- Halothane
- Enflurane
- Isoflurane
- Sevoflurane
- Nitrous oxide

All the inhalational agents except nitrous oxide can cause malignant hyperpyrexia. Suxamethonium can also cause it.

Isoflurane is known to be associated with a 'coronary steal' syndrome.

FLEXOR TENDON INJURIES

23　　D – Zone 4

24　　B – Zone 2

25　　B – Zone 2

The zones of flexor tendon injury are:

Zone 1 – between the distal interphalangeal and proximal interphalangeal joint creases

Zone 2 – between the midpoint of the middle phalanx and distal palmar crease

Zone 3 – between the distal palmar crease and the distal margin of the carpal tunnel

Zone 4 – over the carpal tunnel

Zone 5 – from the proximal margin of the carpal tunnel up the wrist and forearm

Zone 2 is often referred to as 'no man's land' and repairs here often have poor outcomes.

DAY-CASE SURGERY

26 B – Unsuitable for day-case surgery

27 A – Suitable for day-case surgery

28 B – Unsuitable for day-case surgery

The contraindications to day-case surgery are:

- ASA > 2 (the patient in Q28)
- BMI >35 (The patient in Q26)
- Extent of pathology
- No one at home after the procedure
- Lives more than 1 hour away from the hospital
- No access to a phone

URINARY SYSTEM TRAUMA

29   A – Class I

30   D – Class IV

31   C – Class III

Classification of renal trauma:

Class I – renal contusion or contained subcapsular haematoma

Class II – cortical laceration without urinary extravasation

Class III – parenchymal laceration > 1 cm into renal substance without urinary extravasation

Class IV – laceration across corticomedullary junction

Class V – renovascular pedicle injury

Classification of ureteric trauma:

Class I – haematoma or contusion

Class II – laceration with < 50% transection

Class III – laceration with > 50% transection

Grade IV – complete transection with < 2 cm devascularisation

Grade V – complete transection (avulsion) with > 2 cm devascularisation

BURNS

32   C – 8640 ml

33   B – 5400 ml

34   D – 4320 ml

35   E – 17 280 ml

According to ATLS guidelines, the recommended formula for calculating the volume of fluid required for resuscitation following burns is the Mount Vernon or modified Parkland formula. It calculates the volume of fluid required over the first 24-hour period following the burn (TBSA = total body surface area):

$$4 \text{ ml} \times \%\text{TBSA} \times \text{weight (kg)}$$

Half of this fluid should be given in the first 8 hours post-injury and the remainder over the next 16 hours. The recommended fluid is an isotonic crystalloid such as Hartmann's solution or normal saline.

When calculating the TBSA, the 'rule of 9s' is employed. The head and upper limbs represents 9% each, the anterior and posterior torso and each lower limb represent 18% each, and the perineum is the remaining 1%.

The different depths of burns can be estimated from their appearance. Superficial burns have a localised area of pain and erythema, without signs of blistering. Partial-thickness burns involve the epidermis and the dermis and are red, painful and blistered. Full-thickness burns can be white and waxy or red and leathery. They are dry and painless, and involve the epidermis, dermis and subcutaneous tissues.

ANTI-EMETICS

36 C – Ondansetron

37 B – Metoclopromide

38 A – Cyclizine

39 E – Haloperidol

SURGICAL INCISIONS

40   C – McEvedy's

This patient has a femoral hernia which is likely to be strangulated. In this situation an extraperitoneal approach using a vertical incision over the lateral aspect of the lower rectus sheath is most appropriate. From this position the sac can be withdrawn and, if necessary, bowel resescted. In an elective femoral hernia repair a low inguinal incision (Lockwood) can be made.

41   A – Lanz

This patient gives a history consistent with acute appendicitis. For this procedure either a gridiron or Lanz incision could be used, although in a young female patient a Lanz incision is preferred as this is more in keeping with Langer's lines.

42   B – Kocher's

A Kocher's incision is a subcostal incision used for open cholecystectomy.

43   G – Collar

A collar incision is made for a total or subtotal thyroidectomy.

ANATOMICAL RELATIONS

44   A – Artery

The contents of the popliteal fossa are (from deep to superficial): popliteal artery, popliteal vein, tibial nerve, common peroneal nerve.

45   B – Nerve

From lateral to medial, the contents of the cubital fossa are: biceps tendon, brachial artery, median nerve (TAN).

46   C – Vein

At the renal hilum, from anterior to posterior, lie: renal vein, renal artery, renal pelvis and ureter.

47   B – Nerve

The femoral structures lie (from lateral to medial): femoral nerve, femoral artery, femoral vein, Y-fronts (NAVY).

URINARY TRACT INFECTIONS

48   E – *Proteus* spp.

Staghorn calculi occur in strongly alkaline urine. They are usually associated with bacteria that produce urease, which breaks down urea to form ammonia. *Proteus* is the most common of these.

49   D – *Mycobacterium tuberculosis*

HIV patients and other immunocompromised patients are particularly susceptible to tuberculosis. Tuberculosis should always be suspected in patients with sterile pyuria in the absence of any other demonstrable abnormality.

50   F – *Schistosoma haematobium*

Schistosomiasis is endemic to the Middle East, Egypt in particular. The parasite lays eggs in the urinary tract, causing irritation. It can lead to squamous metaplasia, stone disease, or, if left untreated, squamous cell carcinoma.

DYSPHAGIA

51 F – Oesophageal carcinoma

Oesophageal carcinoma is commoner in smokers, in people with increased alcohol intake, oesophageal strictures or certain dietary deficiencies. Symptoms include dysphagia, retrosternal discomfort, chest pain, aspiration pneumonia and recurrent laryngeal nerve palsy. Prognosis is poor as the tumour readily metastasises.

52 G – Pharyngeal pouch

A pharyngeal pouch occurs in a weakness in the inferior constrictor muscle. It is also known as 'Killian's dehiscence'. It is commoner in males and usual features are halitosis (secondary to the retention of undigested food in the oesophagus), recurrent sore throats, regurgitation of undigested food (sometimes eaten days before), aspiration pneumonia and neck swelling. Treatment is by excision of the pouch.

53 A – Achalasia

Achalasia is a dysmotility disorder of the lower oesophagus. It is of unknown pathogenesis but predisposes to carcinomatous change. Barium swallow shows the typical bird's beak appearance, while manometry shows abnormally high intra-oesophageal resting pressure. Treatment is by balloon dilation, Heller's cardiomyotomy or, more recently, injection of botulinum toxin.

INCONTINENCE

54 B – Bladder outlet obstruction

This man has typical symptoms of an enlarged prostate – reduced flow, increased frequency and incomplete emptying. The most likely explanation is bladder outlet obstruction caused by the enlarged prostate with overflow incontinence.

55 D – Neurogenic incontinence

Multiple sclerosis is a common cause of a neuropathic bladder. The absence of voiding urge supports this diagnosis.

56 F – Small bladder capacity

Interstitial cystitis reduces the compliance of the bladder, leading to a smaller bladder capacity. This leads to high filling pressures for the same volume of urine.

57 C – Genuine stress incontinence

Genuine stress incontinence is usually due to lax pelvic floor muscles. This is especially common in multiparous women who have had multiple vaginal deliveries.

58 B – Bladder outlet obstruction

The poor flow and high residual volume of urine indicate bladder outlet obstruction. Gonorrhoea can cause urethral strictures, leading to bladder outlet obstruction in severe cases.

PRE-OPERATIVE INVESTIGATIONS

59   A – ECG

An ECG is required for anyone over the age of 50 likely to have a general anaesthetic. The procedure itself is relatively minor and not likely to involve any major body fluid losses. As the man is otherwise healthy, no other investigations are necessary.

60   G – No investigation required

This patient is a fit and healthy individual under the age of 40. No investigations are required. The chest infection is transient and does not require further investigation, although it would be appropriate to delay surgery until he has fully recovered from his infection.

61   C – ECG + FBC + U&E

ECG + FBC + U&E are the minimum required investigations for anyone undergoing major surgery. Other investigations such as chest X-ray, spirometry and urinalysis should also be considered.

62   D – ECG + FBC + U&E + chest X-ray

The patient is over 65 and on diuretics, both of which are indications for U&E. An FBC is indicated in those over 60, as is a chest X-ray and ECG.

63   B – ECG + FBC

An FBC is indicated in all women. No other blood tests are indicated in adults aged under 60 in the absence of significant past medical history. An ECG is indicated in those over 50.

64   C – ECG + FBC + U&E

A past medical history of hypertension is an indication for ECG. An FBC is indicated as the patient is female. The patient might be on diuretics for the hypertension and U&E is therefore indicated.

TREATMENT OF ULCERS

65   E – Total contact casting

This foot ulcer in a diabetic patient with peripheral neuropathy is likely to be due to a combination of microvascular disease and the neuropathy. Treatment of this type of ulcer is usually based on off-loading the affected area, hence the use of a total contact cast. In addition, tight diabetic control would be helpful.

66   D – Revascularisation

Although this ulcer has many characteristics of a venous ulcer, the ABPI is low. This indicates an arterial element to the ulcer. Compression bandaging in this case would further compromise the circulation. Revascularisation is needed and, if successful, compression bandaging can be undertaken afterwards.

67   A – Compression bandaging

This is a venous type ulcer. The duplex shows good arterial flow, so compression bandaging would be suitable treatment.

68   C – Excision

This history is compatible with malignant change in a chronic ulcer. Surgical excision would be the most appropriate option and skin grafting might be required afterwards.

69   D – Revascularisation

This is an arterial ulcer with stigmata of chronic arterial insufficiency. Revascularisation should be attempted, either endovascularly or surgically.

SURGICALLY IMPORTANT ORGANISMS

70   A – *Acinetobacter*

Acinetobacter is an environmental micro-organism that is resistant to many antibiotics. It often is the cause of outbreaks of multidrug-resistant infection in ICUs. Systemic invasion is common.

71   H – *Staphylococcus epidermidis*

Staphylococcus epidermidis is a commensal of the skin and is normally non-virulent. It is often responsible for infections involving prostheses, either joints or grafts. *Staphylococcus aureus* is coagulase-positive.

72   B – *Bacteroides fragilis*

Bacteroides fragilis is the commonest organism causing serious anaerobic infection. It is particularly common after abdominal or gynaecological procedures. It produces β-lactamase and is therefore penicillin-resistant.

73   D – Fusobacteria

Tonsillar infection is called 'Vincent's angina'. *Fusobacterium fusiformis* and *Borrelia vincentii* are the two usual causes. *Fusobacterium fusiformis* is a Gram-negative rod-shaped organism.

74   F – *Pseudomonas aeruginosa*

Pseudomonas aeruginosa is a Gram-negative bacillus, and is a commensal in human and animal gastrointestinal tracts, water and the soil. It is a common pathogen in immunocompromised patients and those with other underlying pathology. It is resistant to most antibiotics.

CORD LESIONS

75   B – Brown–Séquard syndrome

In this scenario there is hemisection of the cord, resulting in paralysis on the affected side below the lesion, along with loss of proprioception and fine discrimination. Pain and temperature sensation are lost on the opposite side as the spinothalamic tract carries fibres which have decussated at a lower level.

76   E – Posterior cord syndrome

Hyperextension injuries with fractures of the posterior vertebral elements commonly cause posterior cord syndrome. The posterior columns are affected, so proprioception is affected, causing the profound ataxia.

77   A – Anterior cord syndrome

Anterior cord syndrome is common after compression fractures of the vertebral bodies. There is often damage to the anterior spinal artery, so the neurological damage is a combination of direct trauma and ischaemic damage. Corticospinal and spinothalamic tracts are involved, causing loss of power and reduction in pain and temperature sensation below the affected level.

78   D – Central cord syndrome

Central cord syndrome is usually seen in older patients with cervical spondylosis. The cord can be compressed by an osteophyte and intervertebral disc anteriorly and ligamentum flavum posteriorly. This results in flaccid weakness of the arms but preservation of motor and sensory fibres to the lower limb, as these are located more peripherally in the cord.

BENIGN ANO-RECTAL CONDITIONS

79   A – Delorme's procedure

Delorme's procedure involves excising the excess prolapsed rectal mucosa, with the underlying muscle being sutured up in a concertina fashion.

80   B – Diltiazem ointment

Fissure-in-ano is a common condition. Pain on defecation is the most common symptom, and others include pruritus ani, minor bleeding and constipation secondary to pain. It is the most common lesion in Crohn's disease. Treatment is usually medical: either diltiazem cream or glycerol trinitrate ointment. In addition, stool-bulking agents can be used to ease the constipation.

81   F – Rubber-band ligation

This is a classic history of haemorrhoids. They are normally found at the 3-, 7- and 11-o'clock positions in the anal canal. First-line treatment usually consists of rubber-band ligation or injection with sclerosants. Persistent, troublesome haemorrhoids can be treated with haemorrhoidectomy.

82   G – Seton drainage

Inter-sphincteric abscesses can be incised, drained and laid open. Trans-sphincteric abscesses are usually laid open to reduce the risk of incontinence following damage to both internal and external sphincter mechanisms. In this case seton drainage is used, where a suture is tied along the line of the fistula.

PAIN IN THE RIGHT UPPER QUADRANT

83 C – Biliary colic

Biliary colic causes RUQ pain without pyrexia; jaundice is not uncommon if the calculus obstructs the common bile duct.

84 B – Ascending cholangitis

RUQ pain associated with jaundice points to a biliary cause, but the lack of a calculus in the common bile duct rules out cholecystitis.

85 J – Subphrenic abscess

Subphrenic abscess is a known complication of diverticular disease, usually occurring approximately 1–3 weeks following the initial episode.

86 A – Acute pancreatitis

Amylase of >1000 Somorgyi U/dl is characteristic of acute pancreatitis.

87 G – Lower lobe pneumonia

The fact the patient has no rigors and no other signs of disease in the RUQ suggests an infective cause, which can refer pain to the RUQ.

VENTILATORS

88 A – ASB

ASB is a pressure-controlled, flow-cycled mode of ventilation. The patient is required to breathe for themselves in this method. It can be combined with either BIPAP or SIMV to support spontaneous breaths that occur during these modes of ventilation.

89 C – CMV

This is generally reserved for use in operating theatres alone, as it is difficult to wean patients using this method of ventilation only. It operates on either a set volume or a set inspiratory pressure. There is no active patient interaction.

90 D – CPAP

CPAP is one of the simplest forms of ventilation. It uses a face mask and provides a continuous positive pressure. It improves the compliance of the lungs, thereby reducing the work of breathing. It can also help with opening up collapsed alveoli in cases of atelectasis.

91 G – SIMV

SIMV requires the tidal volume and rate to be set, but there is also a time set between each breath during which, if the patient initiates a spontaneous breath, the mandatory breath is synchronised with this. This allows for patient–machine interactivity and the patient can be effectively weaned by increasing the time between each mandatory breath.

MANAGEMENT OF CHEST TRAUMA

92   G – Needle thoracocentesis

This man has signs of a tension pneumothorax. Hyper-resonance, absence of breath sounds and tracheal deviation all support the diagnosis. He has already had a needle thoracocentesis, but during transfer the cannula may have displaced or occluded. A further attempt at needle thoracocentesis should be made. Definitive treatment is with a chest drain.

93   I – Urgent arteriography

This man may have traumatic aortic rupture. The widened mediastinum, left haemothorax and deviation of the trachea to the right support this diagnosis. Although this patient appears stable, it is imperative that further assessment of his aorta is carried out by means of either a CT scan or arteriography. Patients with aortic injury who have a chance of survival usually have an incomplete laceration near the ligamentum arteriosum of the aorta. Specific signs are frequently absent and further investigation is warranted if aortic injury is suspected.

94   D – Immediate open thoracotomy

Patients with penetrating thoracic injuries who present with cardiac arrest or pulseless electrical activity are candidates for immediate open thoracotomy. Closed cardiopulmonary resuscitation would not be effective in this situation. A left anterior thoracotomy is the procedure of choice, with ongoing resuscitation procedures.

CARCINOGENS

95 C – Carcinoma of the bladder

Schistosomes are parasites which invade the urinary tract, and can lay eggs in the bladder. Schistosomiasis is associated with chronic inflammation of the bladder and squamous cell carcinoma of the bladder.

96 C – Carcinoma of the bladder

B-Naphthylamine is converted to the active carcinogen 1-hydroxy–2-Naphthylamine in the liver, but glucuronidation of the compound in the liver offers some protection. In the bladder, glucuronidase unconjugates the molecule and the active carcinogen is concentrated, exposing the urothelium of the bladder to carcinogenic effects.

97 B – Burkitt's lymphoma

Epstein–Barr virus is associated with Burkitt's lymphoma in the presence of malarial infection.

98 E – MALT tumour

There is a link between *Helicobacter pylori* infection and gastric carcinoma, but it has a stronger association with MALT lymphoma. It has been shown that MALT lymphomas sometimes regress with *H. pylori* infection treatment.

99 F – Hepatocellular carcinoma

Aspergillus flavus releases aflatoxins, which occur as dietary contaminants and are associated with hepatocellular carcinoma.

100 H – Oropharyngeal carcinoma

Betel nuts are chewed in parts of Asia as an alternative to tobacco. This is associated with a higher incidence of oropharyngeal carcinoma.

INOTROPES

101 A – Adrenaline

Adrenaline has strong β-adrenergic effects and is mainly used as a bronchodilator in anaphylactic shock.

102 A – Adrenaline

Adrenaline has a propensity to cause arrhythmia. It is for this reason that adrenaline is used in cardiac arrest situations to try to convert a non-shockable rhythm to ventricular fibrillation – which is susceptible to electrical shock.

103 C – Dopamine

Stimulation of dopaminergic receptors leads to increased renal blood flow, hence increased glomerular filtration rate and increased sodium excretion. However, at higher doses, β_1 receptors are also stimulated, causing an increase in heart rate and contractility, and at very high doses (>10 μg/kg per min) dopamine stimulates α_1 receptors causing reduced tissue perfusion and therefore reducing glomerular filtration rate.

104 E – Noradrenaline

Noradrenaline is a powerful α_1 stimulant, and causes strong vasoconstriction. It causes increases in both systolic and diastolic pressure, but also reduces renal blood flow. It is mainly used in the treatment of shock.

SCROTAL SWELLINGS

105 E – Testicular torsion

Testicular torsion usually presents as an exquisitely tender testis, which may be lying horizontally or high-riding. There may be a history of trauma.

106 C – Hydrocoele

Primary hydrocoeles are most common over the age of 40. The swelling fills one side of the scrotum. Fluid collects in the tunica vaginalis, leading to a fluctuant swelling which transilluminates.

107 B – Fournier's gangrene

Fournier's gangrene is necrotising fasciitis of the scrotum. It is caused by a mixed infection in the deep fascia and skin of the perineum, scrotum and penis. Patients can present in septic shock.

TRAUMA

108 E – Intubation

This man has a Glasgow Coma Scale (GCS) of 3. He is unable to protect his own airway; securing the airway is therefore paramount.

109 C – Full spinal and neurological assessment

Calcaneal fractures are high-energy injuries. They are associated with injuries throughout the spinal column, so a full spinal/neurological assessment should be carried out.

110 B – CT scan of the head

This man has a GCS of 11 (eye opening 2, verbal 4, best motor 5). The sudden drop in GCS may indicate an intracranial haemorrhage. A lucid interval such as this is common with extradural haemorrhage and a CT scan is indicated.

LOCAL ANAESTHETICS

111 B – 10 ml

The maximum recommended dose of lidocaine as given in the *British National Formulary* is 200 mg. This equates to 10 ml of 2% lidocaine.

112 D – 30 ml

The maximum recommended dose of bupivacaine as given in the *British National Formulary* is 150 mg. This is equivalent to 30 ml of 0.5% bupivacaine.

113 H – 80 ml

With the addition of adrenaline, the maximum safe dose increases to 200 mg. This equates to 80 ml of 0.25% bupivacaine solution.

114 F – 50 ml

With the addition of adrenaline, the maximum safe dose of lidocaine is 500 mg. This equates to 50 ml of 1% lidocaine solution.

CHEMOTHERAPY

115 C – No chemotherapy

Chemotherapy is usually offered in invasive carcinoma of the breast with lymph node involvement.

116 A – Adjuvant chemotherapy

Currently chemotherapy is offered for all Duke's C carcinomas and Duke's B carcinomas with poor prognostic indicators. These include perforation, vascular invasion and poor differentiation.

117 C – No chemotherapy

Chemotherapy would not be offered in this case as the micrometastases were not detected on routine scanning. Therefore, it would not be possible to monitor response to treatment.

DIAGNOSIS OF ENDOCRINE DISORDERS

118   A – 24-hour VMA

Phaeochromocytomas are tumours of the adrenal medulla arising from chromaffin cells and secrete excess catecholamines. VMA is a breakdown product of catecholamines and therefore urinary levels become elevated.

119   F – Short Synacthen test

Addison's disease is often associated with other autoimmune disorders. It can be investigated for by using the short Synacthen test – this does not cause a rise in plasma cortisol in affected patients whereas it does in unaffected people.

120   C – Plasma aldosterone levels

Diagnosis of Conn syndrome (aldosterone-secreting adrenocortical adenoma) is made by measuring plasma aldosterone, and CT or MRI to locate the adenoma.

121   D – Radio-immunoassay of 17-hydroxyprogesterone

Congenital adrenal hyperplasia occurs as a result of 21-hydroxylase deficiency; 17-hydroxyprogesterone levels are found to be elevated.

122   B – Dexamethasone suppression test

This is a typical presentation of someone with Cushing syndrome. Cushing syndrome can be diagnosed either by measuring 24-hour urinary free cortisol or by an overnight dexamethasone suppression test, which fails to suppress morning cortisol levels in affected patients.

TERMS USED FOR DISORDERS OF GROWTH AND DIFFERENTIATION

123   D – Hyperplasia

Hyperplasia is increased tissue or organ size due to increased cell divisions in response to increased functional demand. This is different from hypertrophy, which is an increase in cell size without replication.

124   B – Atrophy

Atophy is the decrease in size of an organ or tissue by reduction in cell size and/or reduction in cell numbers. It often involves apoptosis and occurs in both pathological and physiological conditions.

125   G – Metaplasia

Metaplasia is the reversible transformation of one type of terminally differentiated cell type. It often occurs in response to environmental stress.

126   A – Agenesis

Agenesis is the failure of development of an organ or structure. This differs from atresia, which is failure of development of a lumen in a normally tubular structure.

CONDITIONS CAUSED BY MICROBES

127 A – *Candida albicans*

Oral candidiasis (thrush) is seen in neonates and immunocompromised patients, or those on long-term antibiotics. It presents as white plaques on the mucous membrane.

128 H – *Streptococcus pyogenes*

Wound infection and surrounding inflammation (cellulitis) is commonly caused by *Streptococcus pyogenes*. This bacterium also causes tonsillitis, otitis media, erysipelas and necrotising fasciitis.

129 D – *Escherichia coli*

E. coli is the causative organism in 90% of community-acquired urinary tract infections and in 50% of hospital-acquired infections. Female diabetics are three times more likely to have a UTI than non-diabetics.

130 C – *Clostridium perfringens*

C. perfringens is a normal bowel inhabitant. However, when present in an anaerobic environment such as a wound, its spores are converted into toxin-producing pathogens. The toxins destroy the surrounding microcirculation. Gas formation occurs, with local crepitus.

131 B – *Clostridium difficile*

C. difficile causes a diarrhoea which is generally associated with broad-spectrum antibiotic use. The best method of diagnosis is the demonstration of specific toxin in the faeces.

132 E – *Helicobacter pylori*

H. pylori is a Gram-negative, spirally shaped bacterium which colonises the gastric mucosa. It can cause gastritis and duodenal ulceration and puts patients at risk of developing gastric ulcers and carcinoma.

HYPERSENSITIVITY REACTIONS

133   D – Type IV hypersensitivity reaction

This type of reaction is also called 'cell-mediated' and is mediated by T-cells which have been sensitised previously by an allergen. They activate cytotoxic T-cells; which recruit and activate macrophages.

134   C – Type III hypersensitivity reaction

This type of reaction is also called 'immune complex–mediated'. It results in the formation of antigen–antibody complexes in the circulation or at extravascular sites, which leads to complement activation, then neutrophil activation.

135   A – Type I hypersensitivity reaction

Type I reactions are also known as 'immediate' reactions. The body forms IgE in response to exposure to a certain allergen. IgE then binds to mast cells and basophils so that when there is re-exposure to the allergen, inflammatory mediators are released from the basophils and mast cells.

136   D – Type IV hypersensitivity reaction

See answer to Q 133.

137   A – Type I hypersensitivity reaction

See answer to Q 135.

138   B – Type II hypersensitivity reaction

Type II reactions are also known as 'cytotoxic' reactions. They are mediated by antibodies formed against antigens. Tissue damage then results via a variety of mechanisms, including complement and antibody-dependent cell-mediated cytotoxicity.

GLASGOW COMA SCALE SCORES

139 E – 10

140 C – 7

141 C – 7

142 F – 13

The Glasgow Coma Scale (GCS) is a system used to record and monitor a patient's level of consciousness. There are a total of 15 points, based on four categories: best motor response (6 = obeys commands; 5 = localises to pain; 4 = withdraws from pain; 3 = abnormal flexion; 2 = abnormal extension; 1 = none), best verbal response (5 = orientated; 4 = confused; 3 = inappropriate speech; 2 = incomprehensible sounds; 1 = none) and best eye-opening response (4 = open spontaneously; 3 = open to speech; 2 = open to painful stimulus; 1 = none). A GCS of 8 is an important score as it is at this point that you consider a patient for intubation as they are unlikely to be able to protect their own airway.

MANAGEMENT OF TRANSITIONAL CELL CARCINOMA OF THE BLADDER

143 G – Nephro-uretectomy

Transitional cell carcinomas of the renal pelvis resemble those affecting the bladder but are much less common. They tend to invade the renal parenchyma and have a tendency to distal spread. There is also a strong tendency for these tumours to be multifocal. Conventional surgical treatment is by nephro-uretectomy and the ureter must be removed with a cuff of bladder wall.

144 C – Cystectomy + urethrectomy + ileal conduit

In patients who have primary CIS which is unresponsive to medical management, cystectomy is an option. Often this is accompanied by urethrectomy as the urethra is often also involved. Urine is commonly diverted into an ileal conduit.

HAEMORRHAGIC SHOCK

145   C – Class III haemorrhagic shock

146   B – Class II haemorrhagic shock

147   C – Class III haemorrhagic shock

Reduction of blood volume is associated with physiological responses mainly mediated by the sympathetic nervous system, which aim to maintain blood pressure and hence blood supply to the vital organs. Haemorrhagic shock can be divided into four classes depending on the amount of blood lost. Each class is associated with particular parameters which help in the estimation of blood loss.

- **Class I** is loss of 0–15% of circulating volume; there are no obvious changes apart from the patient perhaps feeling uncomfortable and restless.

- **Class II** (15–30% loss) is associated with a rise in pulse rate to greater than 100/min, urine output reduced to 20–30 ml/h and a raised RR of 20–30 breaths/min. The BP is normal but pulse pressure is reduced.

- **Class III** (30–40% loss) is associated with a tachycardia of >120/min, reduction in both pulse pressure and BP and reduction in urine output to 10–20 ml/h.

- **In Class IV** (> 40% blood loss) the patient becomes anxious and may be confused. There is tachycardia of >130/min, BP and pulse pressure are low and the patient is anuric. The RR is over 40 breaths/min.

MANAGEMENT OF THYROID DISEASE

148   D – Propylthiouracil

First-line treatment for Graves' disease is carbimazole. In certain individuals it has the unfortunate side effect of agranulocytosis and so propylthiouracil is used instead.

149   D – Propylthiouracil

Propylthiouracil is also the drug of choice in pregnancy as it is protein-bound and therefore less likely to cross the placenta.

150   E – Radio-iodine ablation

Radio-iodide ablation is safe for patients in whom medical management has failed and who are not planning on becoming pregnant during treatment.

151   F – Subtotal thyroidectomy

Surgery for thyroid disorders is carried out for cosmesis, compression symptoms, retrosternal extension and carcinoma.

CAUSES OF JAUNDICE

152 A – Carcinoma of the head of the pancreas

Painless jaundice together with a history of weight loss is strongly suggestive of a malignancy. Together with an obstructive picture (pale stools and dark urine), carcinoma of the head of the pancreas is the most likely diagnosis.

153 B – Gallstones

Jaundice in children with sickle cell disease can be due to red cell haemolysis. However, coupled with episodes of epigastric pain and an obstructive picture, the most likely diagnosis is gallstone obstruction of the common bile duct as pigment bile stones are common.

154 F – Primary liver carcinoma

Sharing of needles among intravenous drug misusers is a serious risk factor for hepatitis B and C, both of which predispose to the development of hepatocellular cancer in later years. Alpha-fetoprotein is a marker for this cancer, although it is also raised in hepatoma.

KNEE INJURIES

155   D – Medial meniscus tear

Tenderness over the joint line following an acute injury is most likely due to a meniscal injury rather than a collateral ligament. Bucket-handle tears of menisci can result in positioning of the torn meniscus between the articular surfaces preventing full extension of the knee.

156   A – Anterior cruciate ligament tear

Anterior cruciate ligament tears result in rapid swelling of the affected knee. This is because the ligament is intra-articular and haemarthrosis can follow a tear. Hyperextension is a classic mechanism by which these tears occur.

TREATMENT OF PROSTATE CANCER

157   E – Surveillance

Curative treatment for prostate cancer can only be offered to those with T_1 and T_2 disease (ie localised). Such patients can be managed by surveillance alone (digital rectal examination (DRE) and regular prostate-specific antigen (PSA) measurements) with further management when they become symptomatic or when the PSA level rises. Radical prostatectomy is usually only offered to those with a life expectancy of > 10 years and is associated with a relatively high level of impotence and incontinence when compared with other treatments.

158   B – Brachytherapy

Localised disease can also be treated with radiotherapy in the form of external beam radiotherapy, which requires the patient to attend hospital on a daily basis for 4–6 weeks, or brachytherapy, which involves the implantation of radioactive seeds into the prostate. For this treatment the prostate must be less than 50–60 grams as the pubic arch can prevent implantation. T_3 and T_4 (locally advanced and metastatic disease) can be treated with hormone manipulation using luteinising hormone-releasing hormone (LHRH) agonist, anti-androgens or orchidectomy.

159   C – External beam radiotherapy

Radiotherapy can be used for symptomatic metastasis and hormone-relapsed cancer.

MANAGEMENT OF ANKLE INJURIES

160   B – Closed reduction and plaster of Paris

If an ankle fracture is stable (ie one malleolus affected or no talar shift), it can be managed perfectly well by closed reduction and plaster cast.

161   C – Open reduction and internal fixation

Unstable fractures (ie those with talar shift, potential for talar shift or associated fibular fracture extending above the tibial plafond) require open reduction and internal fixation.

162   E – Support, NSAIDs and early mobilisation

Ankle sprains should be managed conservatively with analgesia, with or without strapping, and the patient should be encouraged to move the ankle and weight-bear.

COMPLICATIONS OF COLORECTAL CANCER

163 A – Appendicitis

Appendicitis is a complication of caecal carcinoma due to obstruction of the lumen. However, an important differential is perforation and formation of a localised abscess, which can present with the same symptoms.

164 B – Colocolic intussusception

Intussusception typically presents as in this case and the tumour acts as the apex. Half of all adult intussusceptions are due to carcinoma.

165 C – Fistula formation

Direct invasion of a tumour into a neighbouring organ can cause a fistula, eg vesicocolic, rectovaginal or, in the case in the question, fistulation of the transverse colon to the stomach or duodenum.

ABNORMALITIES OF CALCIUM BALANCE

166   C – Hypoparathyroidism

Hypoparathyroidism presents with the symptoms of hypocalcaemia, including paraesthesia, cramps, tetany, circumoral tingling and convulsions. Although most commonly seen post-operatively owing to damage to the parathyroid glands (eg post-thyroidectomy), hypoparathyroidism is also seen after acute pancreatitis, in chronic renal failure and in vitamin D deficiency.

167   F – Tertiary hyperparathyroidism

Primary hyperparathyroidism is most commonly due to a single parathyroid adenoma causing raised levels of PTH and calcium. Secondary hyperparathyroidism is caused by chronic renal failure in response to a low calcium level and is characterised by a low serum calcium and a raised PTH level. Tertiary hyperparathyroidism is also seen in chronic renal failure and is due to the parathyroid gland becoming hyperplastic and secreting PTH autonomously secondary to long-term stimulation.

168   A – Addison's disease

This is a rarer cause of hypercalcaemia. Pigmentation of the buccal mucosa and postural hypotension are typical features.

MANAGEMENT OF BENIGN PROSTATIC HYPERPLASIA

169   H – TWOC and α-blocker

A recent general anaesthetic and opioid-based analgesia causing constipation are two factors which predispose to developing urinary retention post-operatively. Success rates of TWOC in these circumstances are improved by starting an α-blocker 48 hours prior to catheter removal.

170   D – Open prostatectomy

Symptomatic bladder outflow obstruction secondary to BPH for which medical treatment has failed can be treated by surgery – most commonly TURP or open prostatectomy. Morbidity in patients with large prostates is less if they have an open prostatectomy rather than TURP as this reduces the operation time and avoids the excess fluid absorption that can occur during prolonged TURP surgery. Surgery is best avoided in those keen to start a family and remain sexually active, due to the risk of impotence.

171   B – Finasteride

Finasteride is effective in treating BPH associated with prostates > 30 g and has the additional advantage of reducing prostatic bleeding.

WOUND COMPLICATIONS

172   F – Wound dehiscence

Opening of one or any of the layers of the wound is called dehiscence.

173   C – Evisceration

This complete disruption of all the layers of the abdominal wall closure is called evisceration. It is often preceded by a blood-stained watery discharge.

174   A – Abscess

The low-grade pyrexia, fullness of the wound and purulent exudate with pressure suggest an abscess is more likely than an infection.

MANAGEMENT OF HERNIAS

175 A – Conservative management

Umbilical hernias in young children should be treated conservatively as most resolve spontaneously. Surgical repair should be reserved for those children in whom the hernia has not resolved by the age of 3 years and the fascial defect is > 1.5 cm in diameter. They should then undergo a repair similar to the 'vest over pants' Mayo repair used for repair of paraumbilical hernias in adults.

176 F – Repair via high inguinal (Lotheissen) approach

The Royal College of Surgeons recommends the high inguinal approach for elective repair of femoral hernias, except in thin females, where a low crural approach is advised.

177 B – Laparoscopic repair

Laparoscopic repair of inguinal hernias is recommended for the management of bilateral inguinal hernias unless there are any contraindications present.

TREATMENT OF URINARY TRACT INFECTIONS

178 G – Rifampicin

Tuberculous urinary infections present with symptoms of recurrent UTIs, weight loss, fever and night sweats. Mid-stream urine shows sterile pyuria. It is usually secondary to renal tuberculosis. It usually responds to anti-tuberculous drugs, but in cases with advanced renal disease, infection may not subside until the involved kidney and ureter have been removed. Diabetic patients are particularly prone to developing UTIs.

179 F – Oral ciprofloxacin

If uncomplicated and the patient is systemically well the most common cause is *Escherichia coli* infection and this can be treated with an oral antibiotic such as ciprofloxacin or trimethoprim.

180 C – Intravenous co-amoxiclav (Augmentin)

Loin pain, fever and evidence of urine infection should alert you to the possibility of ascending infection causing pyelonephritis. Intravenous Augmentin and hospital admission is required.

POST-OPERATIVE CRITICAL CARE

181   C – Hypovolaemic shock

This patient has an increased pulse, decreased CVP, cardiac output and stroke volume, which is consistent with hypovolaemic shock.

182   D – Neurogenic shock

The decreased pulse is characteristic of neurogenic shock, which also causes a decreased cardiac output with normal CVP and stroke volume.

183   E – Septic shock

The patient has an increased pulse, normal CVP, decreased stroke volume and increased cardiac output, which is consistent with septic shock.

Normal values: CVP = 2–8 mmHg; cardiac output = 5 l/min; stroke volume = 60–130 ml.

SKIN LESIONS

184 B – Bowen's disease

Full-thickness epidermal dysplasia is characteristic of Bowen's disease, which is most common on the lower limbs.

185 E – Lentigo maligna

Change in pigmentation is common in lentigo maligna, and 90% of these occur on the face.

186 J – Squamous cell carcinoma

Squamous cell carcinoma is most common on sun-exposed areas, frequently bleeds and is characterised by an everted edge.

187 A – Basal cell carcinoma

Basal cell carcinoma is characterised by a rolled pearly edge. It does not tend to bleed as often as a squamous cell carcinoma.

ANSWERS
PRACTICE PAPER 2

WOUND CLOSURE

1   F – Free flap

2   A – Healing by secondary intention with simple dressings

3   E – Local flap

4   E – Local flap

5   C – Split-thickness skin graft

6   C – Split-thickness skin graft

Healing by secondary intention with simple dressings is very useful in areas where there is an abundant blood supply, eg the pulp of the finger, and when the wound is small enough and not too deep.

Primary closure is reserved for clean wounds with sufficient margins to be closed without tension; this can be made possible by some undermining of the skin edge.

Split-skin grafting can be used for more extensive wounds and for deeper wounds, but cannot be used to cover exposed bone, cartilage or tendon. It is very useful in burns to cover the defect and prevent further fluid loss. It can be expanded to cover larger defects using mesh.

Full-thickness skin grafting can be used on exposed tendon, but is not good for exposed bone or cartilage.

Local flaps provide their own blood supply and can transfer skin, fascia, muscle and bone if required. They are very useful in areas where the skin is specialised for its function, eg fingers, scalp.

Free flaps also provide their own blood supply and can be used when no local flap is available.

CARDIAC MURMURS

7   C – Aortic stenosis

8   A – Mitral stenosis

9   E – Atrial septal defect

10   G – Patent ductus arteriosus

11   D – Aortic regurgitation

The features of these murmurs:

Mitral stenosis

Dyspnoea, fatigue, palpitations, chest pain, emboli and haemoptysis. Atrial fibrillation (AF) and a malar flush. The apex beat is undisplaced and a mid-diastolic murmur is present.

Mitral regurgitation

Dyspnoea, fatigue, palpitations and AF. The apex beat is displaced and a pansystolic murmur radiating to the apex is present.

Aortic stenosis

Angina, dyspnoea, dizziness, fainting, congestive cardiac failure (CCF). Senile calcification is the commonest cause. The apex beat is undisplaced and an ejection systolic murmur radiating to the carotids is present.

Aortic regurgitation

Dyspnoea, palpitations and cardiac failure. Multiple associated signs including Corrigan's, de Musset's, Quincke's, Duroziez's and Traube's. A water-hammer (collapsing) pulse is associated. The apex beat is displaced and a high-pitched early diastolic murmur is present.

Atrial septal defect

Dyspnoea, CCF and, in infants, failure to thrive. Can present in infancy or adulthood in association with hypertension, commonly aged 40–60 years. AF and a raised JVP. Pulmonary ejection systolic murmur present.

Ventricular septal defect

Can present with severe heart failure in infancy or with dyspnoea and CCF in later life. Harsh pansystolic murmur is present.

Patent ductus arteriosus

Failure to thrive, pneumonia and heart failure. Systolic murmur loudest in the pulmonary area is present.

TREATMENT OF TESTICULAR TUMOURS

12   A – Chemotherapy

Teratomas are less radiosensitive, and therefore localised disease requires orchidectomy and surveillance. Higher stage disease requires chemotherapy.

13   G – Testicular biopsy

Undescended testes have a 20–30-fold greater incidence of developing a tumour. In those who have a previous diagnosis of testicular cancer, the remaining undescended testis should be biopsied.

14   B – Chemotherapy and radiotherapy

Seminomas are very radiosensitive. Stage I and II tumours can be treated by orchidectomy and radiotherapy alone, but further spread requires chemotherapy in addition.

TYPES OF HERNIA

15   D – Littre's hernia

A hernia which contains a strangulated Meckel's diverticulum is known as 'Littre's hernia', and it can progress to gangrene, suppuration and formation of a local fistula.

16   B – Femoral hernia

Hernias that present below and lateral to the pubic tubercle are femoral hernias as opposed to inguinal hernias, which present above and medial to the pubic tubercle.

17   C – Indirect inguinal hernia

Inguinal hernias that can be controlled by pressure over the deep inguinal ring are indirect hernias.

18   E – Lumbar hernia

Hernias which appear spontaneously just superior to the iliac crest are most likely to be lumbar hernias. They occur through the lumbar triangle of Petit, which is formed by the iliac crest, posterior external oblique and anterior latissimus dorsi.

19   F – Paraumbilical hernia

Paraumbilical hernias are more common in men than in women and they are more common in people with COPD, ascites, multiple pregnancies and malignancy. They pass through the linea alba *adjacent* to umbilical cicatrix, as opposed to umbilical hernias, which pass *through* the umbilical cicatrix.

20   G – Spigelian hernia

Spigelian hernias pass through the internal oblique fibres at this level and are also known as 'semilunar line' hernias. They are often defected laterally by the external oblique and felt at the iliac crest. They are more common in women and often cause aching.

21   J – Richter's hernia

Richter's hernia is a complication of hernias, in which the antimesenteric border of the bowel is entrapped. Madyl's hernia is another complication of hernias, in which a W-shaped loop of bowel is trapped and the intervening loop strangulated.

BONE TUMOURS

22   H – Osteosarcoma

Osteosarcoma has a bimodal distribution, with 75% of those affected being aged between 10 and 25 years. The remainder are elderly people with a history of Paget's disease. Osteosarcoma typically presents as a painful mass, most commonly affecting the lower femur and arising from the medullary cavity. It can be a lytic or sclerotic lesion. Those with a history of retinoblastoma have a 5000-fold increased risk of developing an osteosarcoma.

23   B – Chondrosarcoma

Chondrosarcomas can present de novo or as malignant transformation of a benign cartilage tumour such an osteochondroma. They usually affect middle-aged or elderly people.

24   C – Ewing's sarcoma

Ewing's sarcoma usually affects young people aged between 5 and 15 years. It presents as a lytic lesion which causes a periosteal reaction, giving it a characteristic 'onion skin' appearance.

25   H – Osteosarcoma

See answer to Q22.

MANAGEMENT OF ACUTE ISCHAEMIA

26   C – Embolectomy

History of limb ischaemia with no previous chronic symptoms, together with a history of atrial fibrillation, is suggestive of an embolus being the cause of the occlusion. As the history is quite short, embolectomy should be carried out.

27   A – Amputation

A prolonged history of ischaemia means that reperfusion of the limb is hazardous as this can lead to reperfusion injury, which can result in pulmonary oedema, acute respiratory distress syndrome, renal failure and myocardial dysfunction. In such cases amputation is often the safest option.

28   E – Reconstruction

Acute on chronic ischaemia is usually secondary to thrombus formation on the surface of an atheromatous plaque. If sensory or motor deficit is present and run-off is good, a reconstructive operation is advised.

29   A – Amputation

If run-off is poor (with or without thrombus), amputation is recommended. If there is no motor or sensory deficit, thrombolysis is indicated as long as there are no contraindications. If this fails and an angiogram demonstrates poor run-off, amputation should be performed.

NECK LUMPS

30 E – Thyroglossal cyst

Thyroglossal cysts are remnants of the thyroglossal duct, which runs from the back of the tongue to and including the middle third of the hyoid bone. They are midline structures which can be differentiated from thyroid swellings by the fact that they move on protrusion of the tongue.

31 B – Cystic hygroma

Cystic hygromas are congenital cystic lymphatic malformations at the root of the neck which transilluminate.

32 G – Toxic multinodular goitre

Thyroid swellings which feel irregular and are associated with symptoms of hyperthyroidism are likely to be toxic multinodular goitres as thyroid cancers rarely present with toxic symptoms.

33 A – Branchial cyst

A lump appearing between the upper and middle thirds of the sternocleidomastoid in a 35-year-old is most likely to be a branchial cyst, which originates from the remnant of the second branchial arch. It should be excised before it becomes infected.

34 C – Lymph node

A supraclavicular mass together with the symptoms described is highly suggestive of Virchow's node in association with a gastric carcinoma.

35 J – Chemodectoma

Chemodectomas (carotid body tumours) are tumours of the chemoreceptor tissue in the carotid bodies. They arise in the carotid bifurcation at the level of the hyoid bone. There is sometimes a transmitted pulsation from the adjacent arteries, and compression of the arteries can produce symptoms of transient cerebral ischaemia such as blackouts, transient paralysis or paraesthesia.

SURGICAL MANAGEMENT OF INFLAMMATORY BOWEL DISEASE

36   D – Proctocolectomy and ileo-anal pouch

Ulcerative colitis is restricted to the large bowel and is always continuous with a diseased rectum. The traditional approach to eliminate all disease and remove the risk of developing a malignancy is a proctocolectomy and ileostomy formation. In a younger patient, for whom a permanent stoma is unacceptable, an alternative is to form a 'pouch' from the ileum and anastomose this to the dentate line. When the rectum is not involved, a colectomy and ileo-rectal anastomosis avoids a stoma.

37   G – Subtotal colectomy + ileostomy + mucous fistula

Emergency surgery in ulcerative colitis, eg to treat a perforation, is usually managed with subtotal colectomy, ileostomy and mucous fistula. This leaves an intact rectum and anal sphincter for restorative surgery in the future.

38   F – Stricturoplasty

This is a bowel-preserving technique in which inflammatory strictures are incised longitudinally and then sutured transversely, thus widening the bowel wall.

39   C – Ileo-caecal resection

Crohn's disease surgery differs from the management of ulcerative colitis as the purpose is to preserve as much bowel length as possible. Due to its relapsing and remitting nature and tendency to affect any part if the gastrointestinal tract, no surgery can be considered curative.

40   A – Colectomy and ileo-rectal anastomosis

This is used in both Crohn's disease and ulcerative colitis to avoid an ileostomy. Around 33% of patients have a good result and 33% have a poor result – usually due to recurrent disease.

SCROTAL SWELLINGS

41 F – Hydrocoele

A hydrocoele is an abnormal collection of fluid within the tunica vaginalis. It can be primary or secondary to a disease process such as infection or carcinoma. It is fluctuant, transilluminable and it is impossibe to feel the testis as a separate structure.

42 C – Epididymal cyst

An epididymal cyst is a fluid-filled swelling connected with the epididymis which is usually painless. It is fluctuant, transilluminable and felt separate to both the testis and the cord structures. It lies above and slightly behind the testis.

43 D – Chronic epididymo-orchitis

Chronic epididymo-orchitis is most commonly due to TB but can also be caused by sarcoidosis and unresolved acute epididymo-orchitis. Usually presents as a painless hard nodule and can be associated with a hydrocoele or ulceration and sinus formation on the scrotal skin. It may be treated with standard anti-tuberculosis medication.

44 J – Varicocele

A varicocele is 'varicose veins of the spermatic cord' and is due to dilatation of the veins in the pampiniform plexus. It is usually asymptomatic can cause a dragging, aching pain. It is soft, irregularly shaped and non-transilluminable and disappears on lying down. Sudden appearance of a varicocele in older men should alert you to the possibility of retroperitoneal disease.

45 G – Inguino-scrotal hernia

Inguino-scrotal hernias are those which descend into the scrotum and are most commonly of the indirect type. They are soft, reducible and non-transilluminable and it is impossible to get above them, although possible to feel the testis as a separate structure. A cough impulse is present.

46   B – Encysted hydrocoele of the cord

An encysted hydrocoele of the cord is a fluid-filled structure which can lie at any point between the inguinal ring and the upper scrotum. It is fluctuant and transilluminable and it is possible to feel the testis as a separate structure.

UPPER LIMB FRACTURES

47   E – Monteggia's fracture

48   A – Barton's fracture

Monteggia's and Galeazzi's fractures are forearm fractures associated with a dislocation. Monteggia's fracture is a fracture of the upper third of the ulna together with a dislocated radial head, whereas Galeazzi's fracture is a fracture of the shaft of the radius together with a dislocation of the inferior radio-ulnar joint.

49   F – Smith's fracture

50   D – Galeazzi's fracture

Smith's and Colles' fractures are both extra-articular fractures of the distal radius, but in Smith's fracture there is volar displacement of the distal fragment whereas in Colles' fracture there is dorsal and radial displacement. By definition, Colles' fracture must occur within 2.5 cm of the wrist joint. Barton's fracture is an intra-articular fracture of the distal radius associated with subluxation of the carpus.

STAGING OF COLON CANCER

51   C – Duke's C stage

52   C – Duke's C stage

53   A – Duke's A stage

Colorectal cancers are staged primarily on the pathological features of the resected specimen using Duke's system. Clinical staging takes account of whether the resection margin is involved. Staging is as follows:

A = Confined to bowel wall

B = Spread through bowel wall but no nodes involved

C = Lymph node involvement

D = Distant metastases

Stage D was not included in the original staging but is often used. Stage C is often divided into stage C1 (highest node not involved) and stage C2 (highest node involved). Stage is related to 5-year survival rate.

URINARY SYSTEM TRAUMA

54   F – Urethrogram

Blood at the urethral meatus is a strong indicator of urethral rupture. In these circumstances, catheterisation is contraindicated. Urethrography should be performed using water-soluble contrast to demonstrate any leaks and if injury is confirmed, a suprapubic catheter should be sited. Formal urethral repair should be delayed for 3–6 months.

55   E – Surgical exploration

If an injury is sustained to the suprapubic region and bladder trauma is suspected, cystography should be carried out as long as there is no blood at the meatus. Testicular trauma often results in haematoma formation. If this is small with no evidence of testicular rupture, it can be managed conservatively. If the haematoma is large, increasingly painful or there is evidence of testicular rupture, surgical exploration and evacuation of haematoma is required.

56   B – CT scan

Renal trauma is most commonly blunt. In penetrating injuries or those due to rib fractures, associated injuries should be looked for. All such injuries should be investigated by CT scan or high-dose IVU.

PREPARATION OF PATIENTS FOR ENDOCRINE SURGERY

57 G – Vocal cord examination

Patients due to undergo thyroidectomy require vocal cord examination as there is a risk of nerve damage during the operation. They should also be rendered euthyroid to prevent a 'thyroid storm' occurring when the thyroid is handled.

58 E – Thallium technetium scan

Parathyroidectomy should be preceded by a technetium scan. This is because although 80% of primary hyperparathyroidism cases are due to a single adenoma, 10–15% have hyperplasia and 2% have two adenomas. All four parathyroids therefore need to be located because they can occur in a variety of positions from the hyoid bone to the mediastinum.

59 D – Phenoxybenzamine and propranolol

Patients due to undergo adrenalectomy must be thoroughly prepared with α- and β-adrenergic blockade using phenoxybenzamine and propranolol, respectively, as potentially fatal changes in the cardiovascular system can occur under anaesthesia and while handling the tumour.

MANAGEMENT OF PAEDIATRIC DISORDERS

60   F – Ramstedt's pyloromyotomy

The baby has typical presenting features of pyloric stenosis secondary to hypertrophy of the circular pyloric muscles. Aetiology is unknown. It is diagnosed by carrying out a test feed and ultrasound scan. Patients should be adequately hydrated and electrolytes corrected prior to surgery.

61   B – Gastrografin enema

The scenario suggests meconium ileus, which is found in 15% of babies with cystic fibrosis due to highly concentrated meconium which obstructs the terminal ileum pre-natally. This can be diagnosed pre-natally by ultrasound scan. Gastrografin enema can be therapeutic in an uncomplicated case due to its detergent-like effect, which loosens the meconium. However, the baby should also be prepared for laparotomy.

62   D – Laparotomy and proceed

The history is typical of intussusception. First-line treatment is hydrostatic or pneumatic reduction if there no evidence of peritonitis and if it is less than 24 hours since onset. However, if recurrent, laparotomy is indicated to identify a precipitating cause, eg Meckel's diverticulum or a polyp.

RENAL STONES

63 F – PCNL

Stones < 2 cm in the kidney or ureter are generally treated with ESWL. However, this is contraindicated in pregnancy or in patients with abdominal aortic aneurysms (AAAs) which lie in the blast path. In such patients PCNL is a better option. This is also the preferred option for stones > 2 cm or those > 1 cm in the lower pole region as they have poor clearance rates.

64 A – Watch and wait

Stones < 0.5 cm are likely to pass spontaneously unless impacted and so a watch and wait policy is acceptable as long as adequate analgesia is given.

65 B – ESWL (See answer to Q63)

66 F – PCNL

Nephrectomy is the preferred option for treatment of renal calculi if the affected kidney has a differential function of < 15% (with normal global renal function). The presence of infection in an upper urinary tract obstructed by stone is dangerous and is an indication for urgent surgical intervention irrespective of the size of the stone.

67 A – Watch and wait

Indications for conservative treatment of renal calculi include those less than 5 mm diameter, medullary sponge kidney and calculi within cysts.

68 E – Laparoscopic ureterolithotomy

This is a large stone load, and the location of the calculus would require multiple treatments with ESWL, whereas laparoscopic ureterolithotomy allows this to be dealt with in a single procedure.

69 C – Flexible ureteroscopy

The lower pole of the kidney is unfavourable anatomy for ESWL; flexible ureteroscopy is superior.

MANAGEMENT OF THYROID CANCER

70   E – Total thyroidectomy and thyroxine replacement

Papillary carcinoma of the thyroid is often seen in younger patients with a history of irradiation to the neck. Histological examination shows pale, empty-looking nuclei – so-called 'orphan Annie' nuclei. The 10-year survival rate is 90%.

71   D – Surgery and external beam radiotherapy

Elderly patients are more likely to develop anaplastic carcinomas, which have a very poor prognosis despite treatment with surgery and radiotherapy.

72   E – Total thyroidectomy and thyroxine replacement

Medullary carcinomas of the thyroid are tumours of C-cells which produce calcitonin and are associated with familial MEN syndrome.

73   D – Surgery and external beam radiotherapy

Lymphoma of the thyroid is treated in a similar way to anaplastic carcinoma but has better results.

PRURITUS ANI

74   B – Anal fissure

Constipated patients (eg due to opioid-based analgesia) can develop anal fissures – longitudinal tears of the lower half of the anal canal. Although haemorrhoids can also present in this way they are infrequently associated with severe pain unless thrombosed. The pain associated with anal fissures can last for 1–2 hours following defecation.

75   A – Anal carcinoma

Anal carcinoma is more common in homosexuals with a history of anal or genital warts and presents with bleeding, pain, swelling or ulceration and may be associated with enlarged inguinal lymph nodes. Diagnosis should be confirmed with examination under anaesthetic (EUA) and biopsy. Syphilis can present in a similar way but more usually as an shallow ulcer (chancre) rather than a mass.

76   H – Yeast infection

Steroids and other immunosuppressants are used in the medical management of ulcerative colitis and they predispose patients to developing opportunistic yeast overgrowth. Candidal infections affecting the skin usually cause areas of erythema with a well-demarcated edge.

77   D – Fistula-in-ano

Fistula-in-ano can develop de novo or can be associated with Crohn's disease. There is discharge of pus from the external opening.

MANAGEMENT OF VENOUS DISEASE OF THE LOWER LIMB

78   D – Sapheno-femoral ligation

Superficial varicosities can be treated conservatively with support stockings but if increasingly symptomatic (or if patient wishes for cosmetic reasons) surgery is indicated. Long and short saphenous vein incompetences are treated by sapheno-femoral and sapheno-popliteal ligation respectively. Branch varicosities can be treated by stab avulsions.

79   E – Split-skin graft

Debridement and compression bandaging is the usual first-line treatment for venous ulcers, as long as the ABPI is greater than 0.5. Failure to heal after 12 weeks of this treatment is an indication for split-skin grafting, as are ulcers greater than 10 cm^2 in size.

80   G – Systemic antibiotics

Infected ulcers should be managed by taking a swab for culture followed by regular cleaning and dressing – topical antibiotics should be avoided. Surrounding cellulitis, however, is an indication for intravenous antibiotics.

81   B – Elevation and NSAIDs

Thrombophlebitis is best managed with elevation, NSAIDs and support stockings.

ABDOMINAL SIGNS

82   C – Cullen's sign

83   D – Grey Turner's sign

Pancreatitis may be associated with discoloration or bruising around the umbilicus (Cullen's sign) or flanks (Grey Turner's sign). This is due to haemorrhagic pancreatitis with retroperitoneal spread of blood.

84   E – Murphy's sign

Murphy's sign is seen in acute cholecystitis and should not be able to be reproduced in the left upper quadrant. It is caused by the downward movement of the inflamed gallbladder onto the examining hand during examination. Boas' sign is also seen in acute cholecystitis.

85   G – Rovsing's sign

Rovsing's sign is seen in acute appendicitis, when palpation in the LIF reproduces pain in the RIF due to movement of the inflamed parietal peritoneum.

ABDOMINAL INCISIONS

86   G – Pfannenstiel's incision

Pfannenstiel's incision provides excellent access for gynaecological procedures as well as bladder and prostate operations. It can also be used for bilateral hernia repair. In the emergency setting, eg suspected torted ovarian cyst, a midline incision may be more appropriate.

87   E – Midline incision

A perforated duodenal ulcer requires access for oversewing and washout, so an upper midline incision is appropriate.

88   B – Kocher's incision

Kocher's incision is a good incision for cholecystectomy on the left and splenectomy on the right. Laparoscopic cholecystectomy is contraindicated in pregnancy.

89   C – Lanz incision

Access for appendicitis can be via a gridiron or Lanz incision. Lanz's incision is more appropriate in a young woman as it is lower and has a better cosmetic result.

90   H – Rooftop incision

Curative surgery for carcinoma of the head of the pancreas usually involves a pancreaticoduodenectomy (Whipple's operation) and is carried out via a rooftop incision.

FULL BLOOD COUNT

Table 2

	Hb	MCV	WCC count	Neutrophils	Eosinophils	Platelets
A	10.0	120	9.0	6.0	0.1	300
B	7.0	80	8.0	5.0	0.2	250
C	6.0	60	7.0	4.0	0.1	170
D	13.5	90	19.0	16.0	0.1	290
E	22.0	87	5.0	2.5	0.3	350
F	15.0	89	14.0	7.5	4.0	350

91   F

Amoebic dysentery, along with other parasitic infections, results in an eosinophilia. This is also seen with allergic reactions and in asthmatics (type I hypersensitivity reaction).

92   A

Alcoholics are prone to developing megaloblastic anaemia (low Hb, high MCV). This occurs when there is defective synthesis of DNA and delayed mitoses, resulting in a nuclear-cytoplasmic asynchrony. It is usually due to vitamin B_{12} or folate deficiency.

93   D

Chronic corticosteroid use can result in an increased release of neutrophils from the bone marrow storage pool, causing a neutrophilia.

94   C

A person diagnosed with right-sided colon cancer has often had the tumour for a while prior to diagnosis, and therefore has probably had long-standing insidious blood loss via the GI tract. This results in iron deficiency, causing a hypochromatic, microcytic anaemia.

95   B

Haemolytic anaemias, where there is destruction of circulating red blood cells, often results in a normocytic anaemia. In addition, release of bilirubin from red blood cells causes jaundice.

96   E

Polycythaemia rubra vera is a myeloproliferative syndrome which causes increased amounts of erythroid precursors with increased red cell mass. Haematocrit and blood viscosity are also raised, increasing the risk of DVT in these individuals.

SALIVARY GLANDS

97 A – Parotid gland

The parotid gland lies behind the mastoid process, styloid process and ramus of the mandible and has the facial nerve, retromandibular vein, external carotid artery and auriculotemporal nerve running through it. The parotid duct pierces the buccinator muscle to drain opposite the second upper molar.

98 C – Submandibular gland

The submandibular gland is a mixed salivary gland secreting mucous and serous saliva. Its duct enters the floor of the mouth next to the frenulum of the tongue. The sublingual gland lies in front of the anterior border of hyoglossus and medial to genioglossus. It is a mucus-secreting gland and is supplied by the lingual artery.

99 C – Submandibular gland

See answer to Q98.

MANAGEMENT OF HERNIAS

100 D – Urgent hernia repair, ie on an elective list but prioritised over benign conditions

This is a femoral hernia, and as such is likely to strangulate. As there is no evidence of strangulation at present, it does not have to be treated as an emergency, but should be treated as a priority.

101 D – Urgent hernia repair, ie on an elective list but prioritised over benign conditions

Inguinal hernias in children do not necessarily cause strangulated bowel, but an incarcerated inguinal hernia is likely to produce testicular ischaemia. Hence it does not have to be repaired as an emergency, as there are no acute problems, but it should be done urgently.

102 D – Urgent hernia repair, ie on an elective list but prioritised over benign conditions

The short duration of this hernia and the fact that it has become irreducible in such a short time-span mean that repairing this hernia should be a priority. Again there are no signs suggestive of strangulation and so an emergency operation is not necessary.

103 C – Emergency hernia repair

This hernia is showing signs of strangulation – it is red, hot and irreducible. Irrespective of the patient's medical condition, this hernia requires emergency repair. One option might be to attempt to repair it under local anaesthesia.

104 A – Conservative management

This is a small, direct, easily reducible hernia. It is at very low risk of strangulation. It can be treated conservatively as it does not seem to be bothering the patient. This decision can be changed should the hernia enlarge or become symptomatic.

105 B – Elective hernia repair

The site of this hernia and the fact that it can be controlled by occluding the deep inguinal ring reveal it to be an indirect inguinal hernia. These extend into the groin more commonly than other hernias. Asymptomatic indirect inguinal hernias have a low risk of strangulation and therefore elective surgery can be performed.

STATISTICS

106 K – 95%

The specificity is the ability to detect that which is truly negative. It is given by the equation:

Specificity = number of true negatives/(number of true negatives + number of false positives) × 100

In this case: 76/(76 + 4) × 100 = 76/80 × 100 = 95%.

107 I – 80%

The sensitivity is the ability of a test to detect a true positive result. It is given by the equation:

Sensitivity = number of true positives/(number of true positives + number of false negatives) ×100

In this case: 96/(96 + 24) × 100 = 96/120 × 100 = 80%.

108 H – 76%

The NPV is the chance that a condition can be ruled out given a negative result. It is given by the equation:

NPV = (all negative results without condition/all negatives) × 100

In this case: (100 – 24)/100 × 100 = 76/100 × 100 = 76%.

109 L – 96%

The PPV is the chance that a condition is present if identified by a positive test. It is given by the equation:

PPV = (all positive results with condition/all positive results) × 100

In this case: (100 – 4)/100 × 100 = 96/100 × 100 = 96%.

PANCREATIC TUMOURS

110 A – Gastrinoma

Peptic ulceration is a feature of 90% of gastrinomas and 30% of gastrinomas are associated with other endocrine tumours (MEN type I).

111 D – Somatostatinoma

Somatostatinomas are rare tumours derived from pancreatic delta cells. Somatostatin delays gastric emptying and inhibits production of both insulin and glucagons. Clinical features are steatorrhoea, diabetes mellitus and cholelithiasis.

112 B – Glucagonoma

Glucagonomas are tumours of the pancreatic alpha cells. They are rare and can present with an eczematous rash, glossitis, stomatitis, diabetes and weight loss (due to increased gluconeogenesis).

113 I – Zollinger–Ellison tumour

Zollinger–Ellison tumours are rare and affect the non-beta cells of the pancreatic islets of Langerhans. In 90% of cases they present with peptic ulceration; 30% are associated with other endocrine tumours (MEN I).

114 C – Insulinoma

Insulinomas are tumours of the beta cells of the pancreas and are usually solitary. They present with hypoglycaemia.

BREAST INVESTIGATIONS

115   C – Fine-needle aspiration

Even though the lump is clinically and radiologically benign, it is good practice to obtain a cytological diagnosis as part of 'triple assessment'.

116   F – Ultrasound-guided fine-needle aspiration

This woman has a suspicious area on routine mammography. As the area is impalpable it is not possible to do a fine-needle aspiration in clinic, but part of the further investigation of the patient would be an ultrasound scan, and a fine-needle aspiration should be attempted at the same time.

INTRAVENOUS FLUIDS

117   F – Dextran 70

Dextran 70 expands the plasma volume, leading to decreased stasis. It also alters the structure of thrombus to a less organised thrombus, which is supposed to produce smaller, less harmful emboli. However, it is not often used as there is a high risk of anaphylaxis, and it is not as effective as heparin.

118   E – Compound sodium lactate solution

Compound sodium lactate (also known as Ringer's lactate or Hartmann's solution) is the fluid of choice for initial resuscitation according to ATLS guidelines.

119   E – Compound sodium lactate solution

Compound sodium lactate is the only one of the given fluids to contain potassium. It also contains 130 mmol sodium, 111 mmol chloride and 29 mmol lactate.

120   B – 0.9% Sodium chloride solution

0.9% Sodium chloride solution contains 150 mmol sodium; 0.45% sodium chloride solution contains 75 mmol sodium; and 4% dextrose/0.18% sodium chloride contains 30 mmol sodium. Compound sodium lactate contains 131 mmol sodium.

121   D – 5% Dextrose solution

Water tends to follow the sodium ions, so any fluid containing sodium is more likely to remain in the intravascular compartment. The dextrose in any solution is rapidly metabolised, it is the same as giving water. This is spread throughout body fluid, ie intracellular and extracellular fluid, so less remains in the intravascular compartment.

SPECIFIC TESTS

122 C – Lachman's test

Traumatic haemarthrosis is usually caused by anterior cruciate ligament (ACL) rupture, tibial spine avulsion or meniscal tears. The mechanism suggests an ACL injury. Although the pivot shift test would also identify a torn ACL, it is not recommended in clinic with an anxious patient as it can be very painful.

123 B – Froment's test

Froment's test involves asking the patient to hold a piece of paper between the index finger and an adducted thumb. The clinician pulls the paper away. If an ulnar nerve palsy is present, the patient will be unable to adduct the thumb due to paralysis of adductor pollicis. Instead the thumb will flex at the interphalangeal joint due to the action of flexor pollicis longus, which is supplied by the anterior interosseous branch of the median nerve.

124 E – Simmonds' test

The most likely diagnosis in this instance is an Achilles' tendon rupture. Simmonds' test involves asking the patient to kneel facing away from you. Squeezing the calf should produce plantar flexion at the ankle joint. Lack of plantar flexion is indicative of an Achilles' tendon rupture.

CALCULI

125   C – Calcium phosphate

Staghorn calculi form in strongly alkaline urine. They are associated with urinary tract infections with urease-forming bacteria such as *Proteus*. They are composed of magnesium ammonium phosphate with calcium.

126   A – Bile pigment stone

Only 10% of gallstones are radio-opaque and these tend to be composed of calcium bilirubinate. They are associated with chronic haemolytic disease causing excess bilirubin release.

127   B – Calcium oxalate

Calcium oxalate is the most common substance in urinary tract calculi, accounting for approximately 75% of cases.

TYPES OF ULCER

128 C – Cushing's ulcer

Cushing's ulcer is a stress ulcer which occurs secondary to head injury.

129 F – Marjolin's ulcer

The recent changes, the increased vascularity of the ulcer and the rolled edges, suggest malignant change. A squamous cell carcinoma occurring in a chronic venous ulcer is known as 'Marjolin's ulcer'.

130 G – Rodent ulcer

Rodent ulcers (also known as basal cell carcinomas) usually arise on sun-exposed areas of the skin. They classically have raised edges with a pearly white appearance.

131 B – Curling's ulcer

Curling's ulcer is a stress ulcer associated with burns.

SKIN LESIONS

132 B – Dermatofibroma

This has all the characteristics of a benign lesion (slow growing, smooth and small). It is a dermatofibroma (also known as histiocytoma). A dermatofibroma usually occurs on a limb in middle-aged people. It starts as a hemispherical lump which flattens into a disc. It is usually covered by normal-looking skin and has no associated features.

133 H – Strawberry naevus

Strawberry naevi are present from birth. They are usually sessile hemispheres, but as they grow they can become pedunculated. They are compressible but not pulsatile and most common on the head and neck. They can bleed and become ulcerated if knocked.

134 A – Basal cell carcinoma

This is a rodent ulcer or basal cell carcinoma. It is locally invasive, but rarely metastasises. The incidence increases with age as it is related to ultraviolet light exposure. For the same reason it most commonly occurs on the face, above a line drawn from the angle of the mouth to the lobe of the ear. The raised pearly edge is characteristic.

135 D – Melanoma

This is a melanoma. By definition there is no benign melanoma and the presence of a brown halo and jaundice indicates metastatic spread. The majority develop in people between 20 and 30 years of age, and they are more common in whites. They often itch but are rarely painful.

136 F – Pyogenic granuloma

Pyogenic granulomas are an overgrowth of granulation tissue and usually form after a minor insult such as a scratch or small cut. They are most common on the hands and face. They grow rapidly but rarely to more than 1 cm as they outgrow their blood supply.

137   C – Keratoacanthoma

A keratoacanthoma is a self-limiting overgrowth of a hair follicle. The central plug is made up of keratin, and it usually presents as a rapidly growing lump that may begin to regress by the time the person attends clinic. The lump is generally confined to the skin and is mobile over subcutaneous tissue. It can be mistaken for a squamous cell carcinoma due to its rapid growth.

AIRWAY MANAGEMENT

138 H – Single-lumen uncuffed endotracheal tube

The soot in the nasal passages and the respiratory distress suggest a smoke inhalation injury. Early intubation is recommended, and uncuffed tubes are used in children to minimise the chance of tracheal damage.

139 B – Double-lumen cuffed endotracheal tube

A general anaesthetic will be required, hence a definitive airway with endotracheal intubation. A double-lumen tube is used in thoracic surgery so that one lung can be deflated, allowing better access to the chest.

140 D – Needle cricothyroidotomy

It is likely that there is an airway obstruction, and as this man is in respiratory arrest, urgent intervention is required. Percutaneous tracheostomy is time-consuming so needle cricothyroidotomy should be attempted. This is a temporising measure and will allow sufficient ventilation for approximately 30 minutes.

141 F – Percutaneous tracheostomy

Tracheostomy reduces the work of breathing, which improves the chances of weaning the patient from mechanical ventilation. It is also better tolerated and leads to a reduction in inotropes or vasopressors.

142 G – Single-lumen cuffed endotracheal tube

This man again has evidence of smoke inhalation with his nasal hair singeing. A high respiratory rate and reduced oxygen saturation indicate respiratory distress, and as such he requires endotracheal intubation. A single-lumen cuffed tube is most commonly used.

COLORECTAL CARCINOMA PROCEDURES

143   E – Hartmann's procedure

In the acute setting with a patient who has the potential to become extremely unwell through peritonitis, a quick and safe operation is required. Hartmann's procedure involves forming a colostomy and excising the rectum, oversewing the distal end. There is a possibility of reversal once the patient has sufficiently recovered.

144   F – Right hemicolectomy

A right hemicolectomy is performed to excise the tumour and the colon which has the same blood supply from the superior mesenteric artery.

145   A – Abdomino-perineal resection

This is a low rectal tumour and for complete excision it would be hazardous and difficult to maintain the sphincter mechanism. Abdomino-perineal resection is the operation of choice, and in this procedure the colon and rectum are excised from the intraperitoneal and perineal ends.

146   F – Right hemicolectomy

Appendiceal carcinoma is an indication for right hemicolectomy.

147   F – Right hemicolectomy

This is a good story of presentation of a caecal tumour. A right hemicolectomy should be performed.

148   E – Hartmann's procedure

Although anterior resection is possible, in this instance, with the co-morbidities present, a quick operation is essential and it would be better to avoid anastomoses. Hartmann's procedure is therefore the procedure of choice.

149 D – Extended right hemicolectomy

The location of this tumour requires greater resection than a standard right hemicolectomy allows.

150 G– Sigmoid colectomy

This sigmoid lesion requires sigmoid colectomy.

151 B – Anterior resection

Non-obstructing, high rectal tumours are suitable for anterior resection.

THE LIMPING CHILD

152   E – Septic arthritis

The child is septic, with raised inflammatory markers. The diagnosis is septic arthritis of his right hip and he needs a washout of the hip.

153   F – SUFE

SUFE is associated with hypogonadism and is said to occur in short-statured children. It is more common in males. The most common examination finding is restricted internal rotation.

154   A – DDH

Common pathologies at this age include septic arthritis, DDH and irritable hip. Although babies are screened for DDH, as well as some still present at a later age. It is more common in females, associated with congenital foot abnormalities and breech deliveries as well as with first-born children and multiple deliveries.

155   D – Perthes' disease

Perthes' disease is avascular necrosis of the femoral head, which is most commonly seen in boys aged 5–7 years. The radiological changes are usually well established at presentation.

STERILISATION

156   D – Steam sterilisation – 15 minutes at 121 °C

Autoclaving or steam sterilisation is most often used to sterilise surgical instruments. Autoclaves operate at either a cycle of 121 °C for 15 minutes or 134 °C for 3 minutes. This is effective against bacteria, spores and viruses.

157   A – Glutaraldehyde 2%

Colonoscopes require fast turnaround times and repeated use. Therefore 2% glutaraldehyde is used as it is cheap, efficient, fast and easy to use.

158   C – Irradiation

Single-use items which are commercially produced are usually irradiated for sterilisation. This is effective and efficient for large-scale use.

CONSENT

159 A – Accept wishes for non-treatment

Although this man has a chronic mental health problem, he still retains the capacity to make an informed decision about his treatment. He understands that he is likely to die without surgery and his wishes must be respected. Although you may be able to section him under the Mental Health Act, this only allows for treatment of his mental health problem and not for treating the intra-abdominal perforation.

160 C – Proceed to treat without consent of patient

A 13-year-old may be 'Gillick competent' in that if he or she understands the implications and possible complications of treatment, they may consent to that treatment without the express permission of their parents. However, in this instance the child would not be allowed to refuse treatment, as this is not covered by Gillick competence. Parental consent has been obtained, and you can proceed to treat without the consent of the child.

161 C – Proceed to treat without consent of patient

This patient has known dementia and so does not have the capacity to make an informed decision with regard to treatment options. To proceed to operative treatment of the fracture would be to act in the patient's best interests.

162 A – Accept wishes for non-treatment

A signed, witnessed advance directive must be respected. As such, even though the current situation does not relate to the probable cause for the advance directive, the patient's wishes must be respected.

UROLOGICAL INVESTIGATIONS

163 F – Transrectal ultrasound

A raised PSA (upper limit at this age of around 4.5) and a craggy prostate are suspicious of malignancy. Transrectal ultrasound is the imaging of choice, as CT and MRI have not been shown to reliably demonstrate the prostate. It is also imperative to obtain tissue to confirm the diagnosis and to stage the tumour; this can be attempted at the time of the ultrasound.

164 A – Abdominal ultrasound

This man is not producing urine. He has been catheterised adequately, as some urine was obtained, so he must be either dehydrated or have bilateral ureteric obstruction. Pelvic lymphadenopathy from metastatic carcinoma of the prostate does cause this, and an urgent ultrasound scan is indicated to see whether there is any hydronephrosis.

165 A – Abdominal ultrasound

Transabdominal ultrasound is the radiological investigation of choice for frank haematuria as it is safe, non-invasive and good at differentiating solid and cystic masses.

166 A – Abdominal ultrasound

The left testicular vein drains into the left renal vein, whereas the right testicular vein drains directly into the inferior vena cava. A left-sided varicocele therefore raises the possibility of a left renal vein thrombus, which is commonly caused by left-sided renal tumours. An abdominal ultrasound scan is the first-line investigation.

ARTERIAL BLOOD GASES

167   F – Metabolic alkalosis

Metabolic alkalosis: there is a raised pH with increased bicarbonate and a normal $Pa(co_2)$. The normal $Pa(o_2)$ indicates that the respiratory system has not begun to compensate. This situation has arisen due to fluid loss caused by vomiting.

168   A – Compensated metabolic acidosis

Compensated metabolic acidosis: the pH is reduced with decreased bicarbonate. The respiratory compensation lowers the $Pa(co_2)$ and increases the $Pa(o_2)$. This patient has diabetic nephropathy, the chronic nature of which has allowed compensation by the respiratory system.

169   G – Respiratory acidosis

Respiratory acidosis: the pH is reduced, with a raised $Pa(co_2)$ and a normal bicarbonate. In this situation over-sedation is a possible cause. Her poor respiratory effort has caused a reduction in her $Pa(o_2)$.

OBSTRUCTIVE JAUNDICE

170   C – Carcinoma of the pancreas

In the presence of jaundice with a palpable gallbladder, the cause of the obstruction is unlikely to be stone disease and more likely to be a malignancy. In addition, the dilatation of the bile ducts with no visible stone disease supports this diagnosis. Ultrasound does not pick up all pancreatic tumours; CT scanning is more sensitive.

171   G – Sclerosing cholangitis

The steatorrhoea and jaundice are consistent with obstructive jaundice. Sclerosing cholangitis is associated with inflammatory bowel disease, in particular ulcerative colitis, which co-exists in approximately 70% of patients.

172   F – Chronic pancreatitis

The history is typical of pancreatitis, and the recurrent episodes suggest the chronic nature of the disease. In severe cases of chronic pancreatitis, the serum amylase does not necessarily rise, as the cells producing the amylase are destroyed by the disease process.

173   B – Biliary colic

This history is typical of biliary colic. The pain settles as the stone is passed and the obstruction is relieved.

STAGING OF TUMOURS

174   B – Breslow's staging

There are two staging systems for melanomas: Clark's staging is defined by invasion of anatomical layers of the skin, whereas Breslow's staging is based on the depth of invasion. In this instance we only know the depth of invasion, so Breslow's is used.

175   A – Ann Arbor staging

The presence of Reed–Sternberg cells indicates Hodgkin's lymphoma. This is staged using the Ann Arbor staging system.

176   E – Gleason's score

Prostate carcinoma is staged using Gleason's scoring system.

LOWER LIMB NEUROPATHY

177   A – Common peroneal nerve

The common peroneal nerve is in danger of compression when applying below-knee casts. It is vulnerable around the neck of the fibula. Both branches of the peroneal nerve are therefore affected, compromising dorsiflexion (deep peroneal nerve) and eversion (superficial peroneal nerve).

178   F – Sural nerve

The sural nerve is a cutaneous sensory branch of the tibial nerve. It runs just posterior to the short saphenous vein in the leg, so is vulnerable to damage during avulsion of this vein.

179   D – Sciatic nerve

The sciatic nerve is particularly vulnerable in fracture dislocations of the hip. Damage to the nerve has been reported in up to 16% of cases. The quadriceps is spared as it is supplied by the femoral nerve, and its cutaneous branch, the saphenous nerve, supplies sensation to the upper calf and medial aspect of the leg.

180   C – Saphenous nerve

The long saphenous vein is the most commonly used vein for vein grafting procedures. The saphenous nerve runs in close proximity to the vein, supplying the upper calf and medial aspect of the leg. It is vulnerable to damage when the vein is stripped, particularly if it is stripped below the knee.

ANSWERS
PRACTICE PAPER 3

OBSTRUCTION

1   D – Volvulus

A history of constipation and laxative abuse are linked to an increased risk of sigmoid volvulus.

2   E – Carcinoma

A history of altered bowel habit and weight loss associated with obstruction is carcinoma until proved otherwise.

3   A – Paralytic ileus

Ileus is common in post-op patients lying still in bed for lengthy periods and in patients undergoing spinal surgery.

4   G – Gallstone ileus

While previous abdominal surgery predisposes to adhesions, the past medical history of abdominal pain could represent gallstones, and a finding of air outlining the biliary tree or gallbladder on X-ray is characteristic of gallstone ileus.

INVESTIGATION OF RENAL TRAUMA

5   F – Urethrogram

6   H – CT scan with contrast

7   H – CT scan with contrast

8   E – Cystogram

The imaging of renal trauma is dependent on the injury suspected. Plain X-rays, KUB studies and USS have little or no role to play. IVU can be useful for renal injuries, but contrast CT is more sensitive and specific. IVU is used for ureteric injuries, unless other injuries are suspected, in which case contrast CT can image these as well. If blood is seen at the external urethral meatus or there is a high-riding prostate then a urethrogram must be performed prior to catheterisation. In cases of suspected bladder injury a cystogram is the investigation of choice.

The patient in Q5 has blood at the external urethral meatus, so urethrography must be the first investigation, prior to passing a catheter.

The patient in Q6 is most likely to have a renal injury, given the level of the concurrent rib fractures and so contrast CT is required in this stable patient.

The patient in Q7 is likely to have a ureteric injury as over 90% of these are due to penetrating injuries. In light of the risk of other intra-abdominal injuries, contrast CT is preferable to IVU.

Bladder trauma is commonly associated with pelvic fractures and is not well visualised on CT, so cystography is the investigation of choice in the patient in Q8.

BURNS

9   G – 19%

10   C – 2.5%

11   J – 45%

12   D – 9%

The percentage surface area of burns is calculated using Wallace's rule of 9s. Simple areas of erythema (as in question 12) are not included. The percentages for each body part are:

- Head and neck – 9%
- Trunk – 36% (18% anterior aspect and 18% posterior aspect)
- Perineum – 1%
- Arms – 9% each
- Palm of the hand – 1.25%
- Legs – 18% each (9% anterior surface and 9% posterior)

STATISTICS

13 D – Nominal data

14 A – Quantitative measured data

15 C – Ordinal data

Quantitative data: a measurement of how much of a particular variable there is, or how much its respective value is. Measured quantitative data are used for continuous variables, eg BP, and counted quantitative data are used for whole numbers, eg the prevalence of a condition.

Ordinal and nominal data are subtypes of categorical data, which measure the type of the variable. Ordinal data consist of ordered categories, eg staging of cancers, and nominal unordered categories, eg blood groups.

DRAINS

16   D – No drain required

Routine drainage is not recommended following uncomplicated bowel anastomosis.

17   B – Closed suction drain

A closed suction drain is recommended immediately following thyroidectomy to prevent haematoma formation and airway compromise.

18   E – Sump drain

A high-output enteric fistula requires a sump drain to allow both aspiration and irrigation without stimulating further output, and to prevent fistula effluent spilling onto the skin.

19   B – Closed suction drain

A skin flap requires a closed suction drain to prevent haematoma formation disrupting the blood supply to the flap.

20   F – T-tube

T-tubes can be used for CBD (common bile duct) and for oesophageal perforations to prevent further damage to friable tissues.

FRACTURE CLASSIFICATIONS

21 C – Gustilo–Anderson classification

Open fractures are classified using Gustilo–Anderson classification.

22 D – Mason's classification

Mason classified radial head fractures.

23 F – Salter–Harris classification

A distal radial fracture in a child would extend into the epiphysis and is therefore a growth plate injury. These are classified by the Salter–Harris classification.

24 B – Garden's classification

Intracapsular hip fractures are classified using Garden's classification.

LOCAL ANAESTHETICS

25   D – Lidocaine

Lidocaine without adrenaline is the choice of local anaesthetic as the procedure requires rapid onset of anaesthesia. As it is on a digit, adrenaline must not be used.

26   F – Prilocaine

Prilocaine is the most commonly used local anaesthetic for intravenous administration in Bier's blocks.

27   E – Lidocaine and adrenaline

The scalp is very vascular, so adrenaline is used to prevent excessive haemorrhage.

28   A – Bupivacaine

Bupivacaine alone allows longer-duration analgesia once the patient has recovered following a general anaesthetic. Again, adrenaline should not be added as the procedure is on a digit.

29   A – Bupivacaine

Bupivacaine without adrenaline can be used in spinal anaesthesia.

TREATMENT OF FRACTURES

30 D – Open reduction and internal fixation

This type of fracture is an unstable injury which requires an anatomical reduction, and open reduction and internal fixation is necessary to achieve this.

31 A – Broad arm sling

This type of fracture requires treatment only to rest the affected part, and the sling provides relief from the pain.

32 B – Intramedullary nail

This patient has undergone polytrauma, and therefore the fractures need to be treated surgically, so the femoral shaft fracture should be treated with an intramedullary nail, rather than a Thomas' splint.

33 A – Broad arm sling

An undisplaced clavicle fracture with no neurovascular or skin complications requires only conservative treatment, and a broad arm sling is the best of the options.

THE LIMPING CHILD

34 B – Perthes' disease

Perthes' disease is the most likely diagnosis as it is most common in boys aged 5–7 years who are small for their age. The pain tends to be vague and they can have had similar previous episodes.

35 E – Transient synovitis

Transient synovitis is a diagnosis of exclusion, and it is always important to rule out septic arthritis. In this case the child is systemically well, with a recent history of viral illness and normal bloods, as well as loss of internal rotation, making this diagnosis most likely.

36 C – Septic arthritis

Septic arthritis is the most likely cause in this child, as there is a source for haematological spread of infection, the child is systemically unwell and there is pain on all movements.

37 D – SUFE

SUFE is more common in boys aged 14–16 years who are overweight. It tends to present with knee pain and causes loss of abduction.

FRACTURED NECK OF FEMUR

38 E – Thompson's hemiarthroplasty

This patient requires a hemiarthroplasty as the fracture is displaced and intracapsular because avascular necrosis is a significant risk. As the patient does not have significant past medical problems restricting the length of anaesthetic, a cemented (Thompson's) hemiarthroplasty would be the better choice.

39 D – Immediate cannulated screws

This patient is under the age of 65 years with no significant co-morbidities and a minimally displaced intracapsular fracture, so cannulated screws as a surgical emergency are the best choice to preserve the blood supply to the femoral head.

40 C – Dynamic hip screw

This is an inter-trochanteric fracture, so the blood supply to the femoral head is not at risk, and a dynamic hip screw is the most suitable treatment.

41 G – Open reduction and internal fixation

Undisplaced subcapital fractures have a good chance of maintaining the blood supply if there is minimal disruption of the capsule. They can generally be treated with the insertion of cannulated screws. In a displaced fracture (ie Garden III and IV) there is a high risk of developing avascular necrosis of the femoral head, so hemiarthroplasty is the preferred management. The exception is in young patients, for whom preservation of their own femoral head rather than insertion of a prosthesis at a young age is a better option. In such circumstances open reduction and internal fixation is preferable.

42 G – Open reduction and internal fixation

Subtrochanteric extension of the fracture renders it highly unstable, and therefore unsuitable for a dynamic hip screw. It requires open reduction and internal fixation, eg with an intramedullary hip screw.

ISCHAEMIC LIMBS

43   G – Embolectomy

The patient is in atrial fibrillation, which is the most likely cause of the embolus in this previously asymptomatic individual.

44   D – Angiogram and thrombolysis

CCF is a known exacerbating condition for thrombus formation, and the patient is likely to have been relatively immobile.

45   A – Amputation

This is a picture of a patient with chronic arterial insufficiency and acute deterioration. The disease is distal and there is already extensive skin loss and infection, so bypass is not likely to be an option.

46   I – Reconstruction

Acute on chronic ischaemia is usually secondary to thrombus formation on the surface of an atheromatous plaque. If the sensory or motor deficit is present and run-off is good, a reconstructive operation is advised.

ABDOMINAL AORTIC ANEURYSMS

47   G – Ultrasound in 1 year

Annual surveillance is suitable for aneurysms smaller than 4 cm.

48   D – Elective open repair

The gradual increase in size of this aneurysm necessitates an elective repair in a medically fit patient. This aneurysm is unsuitable for endoluminal repair as it is only 0.5 cm below the renal arteries (it would need to be 2 cm below for endoluminal repair).

49   F – Ultrasound in 6 months

The aneurysm is asymptomatic and between 4.0 cm and 5.5 cm, so surveillance should be increased to 6-monthly.

50   E – Urgent elective repair

This rapid increase in size of more than 1 cm means that urgent surgery is required.

CAROTID ARTERY DISEASE

51   B – Endarterectomy left side

The symptom of facial drooping occurs on the contralateral side, and a stenosis of greater than 75% warrants surgical intervention.

52   C – Endarterectomy right side

Visual loss is a symptom which occurs on the ipsilateral side and therefore the right side is responsible for these symptoms.

53   A – Best medical therapy

Hemiparesis is a sign which occurs on the contralateral side, but the stenosis on the right side is 100%. Collateral flow is sufficient as the symptoms resolved, so surgery is not required.

54   A – Best medical therapy

The symptoms suggest a source in the vertebrobasilar territory, not the carotid, so carotid surgery is not indicated.

HEAD INJURIES

55   C – Home with advice

Post-traumatic amnesia and brief loss of consciousness are not indications for admission, and this patient has someone to accompany him home and observe him.

56   A – Admission for neurological observations

This patient requires admission for observation as he is on anticoagulants. Intoxication and clotting abnormalities are also indications for admission.

57   E – Referral to neurosurgery

A depressed skull fracture is an indication for a neurosurgical consultation.

58   B – CT scan

The left haemotympanum suggests a basal skull fracture, and a CT scan is needed to confirm this diagnosis.

BLOOD GAS ANALYSIS

59   D – Metabolic alkalosis

The pH is increased, showing alkalosis. The positive base excess and raised bicarbonate indicate a metabolic cause.

60   E – Metabolic acidosis with compensation

The pH is decreased, indicating acidosis. The decreased bicarbonate and negative base excess indicate that the cause is metabolic. The decreased $Pa(co_2)$ reveals the respiratory compensation.

61   B – Respiratory acidosis with compensation

The pH is decreased, indicating acidosis. The raised $Pa(co_2)$ indicates a respiratory cause and the increased bicarbonate with a normal base excess indicate metabolic compensation.

62   F – Metabolic acidosis without compensation

The pH is decreased, indicating acidosis. The decreased bicarbonate and negative base excess indicate a metabolic cause. The normal $Pa(co_2)$ indicates a lack of respiratory compensation.

CONSENT

63   C – Patient's refusal is valid and doctor cannot override

An adult patient who understands the risks and benefits of the surgery but does not consent cannot be forced to undergo the procedure.

64   B – Patient can give valid consent

A patient younger than 16 years of age, who understands the procedure and its risks and benefits is Gillick competent and can give consent to treatment.

65   A – Doctor can consent for the patient

No adult can consent for another adult, so the daughter cannot consent for her mother. The decision regarding surgery lies with the doctor.

66   B – Patient can give valid consent

A patient under 16 years of age with five GCSEs is likely to be Gillick competent. If the doctor considers him Gillick competent he can consent for himself.

SCROTAL SWELLINGS

67 D – Hernia

Since the swelling cannot be got above and transmits a cough impulse the most likely diagnosis is a hernia.

68 A – Epididymal cyst

As the swelling is separate from the testis but not generalised, this suggests it is in the epididymis and transillumination suggests that it is cystic.

69 E – Hydrocoele

Swelling that cannot be localised to the testis or epididymis and transilluminates points to a hydrocoele.

70 B – Epididymo-orchitis

The epididymis alone being tender, normal lie of the testis, and previous urinary symptoms and systemic symptoms point to epididymo-orchitis rather than torsion in this case.

71 G – Testicular torsion

The sudden-onset severe pain and severe testicular tenderness point to torsion. The normal lie of the testis does not rule this out.

TUMOUR MARKERS

72   E – CEA

CEA is a non-specific tumour marker which can be used for colorectal carcinoma.

73   E – CEA

CEA can also be used as a marker for breast cancer.

74   C – CA 125

CA 125 can be used as a marker for ovarian cancer.

75   J – PSA

PSA can be used for prostate cancer.

76   H – hCG

β-hCG can be used for choriocarcinoma.

77   A – ACTH

ACTH is secreted by small-cell lung cancers.

CONGENITAL GASTROINTESTINAL ANOMALIES

78   C – Gastroschisis

The intestine protruding to the right of the umbilicus points to the diagnosis of gastroschisis instead of exomphalos. Also, in exomphalos the intestine has a membranous covering. The ovaries are more commonly involved in gastroschisis.

79   D – Hirschsprung's disease

The failure to pass meconium, with bilious vomiting and abdominal distension lead to a diagnosis of meconium ileus or Hirschsprung's. The temporary relief of symptoms by removal of the mucus plug make the diagnosis of Hirschsprung's much more likely.

80   H – Small-bowel atresia

That the baby has passed meconium rules out meconium ileus and Hirschsprung's. The X-ray finding of distended bowel points to small-bowel atresia as opposed to duodenal atresia.

81   A – Duodenal atresia

The double bubble sign on the abdominal X-ray is a feature of duodenal atresia, as there is a gastric bubble and a second duodenal bubble. This condition is linked to Down syndrome.

82   E – Hypertrophic pyloric stenosis

The fact that the child was healthy for the first month and then developed the projectile vomiting, and that the feed is unaltered point to pyloric stenosis, which is more common in males.

TREATMENT OF GALLSTONES

83   D – Low-fat diet

The patient is asymptomatic, and only a small proportion of asymptomatic calculi actually go on to provoke an attack or require surgery, so prophylactic surgery is not required.

84   E – Urgent cholecystectomy

In this case the patient is having an acute attack of cholecystitis and may have an empyema, which has failed to settle with conservative treatment, and urgent surgery is required.

85   B – Elective open cholecystectomy

This patient has had several attacks of biliary colic, and therefore requires surgery. However, he has had previous upper abdominal surgery so an open procedure is required.

CHEST INJURIES

86   C – Diaphragmatic rupture

The decreased bowel sounds audible in the left side of the chest point to diaphragmatic rupture. This condition is more common on the left, the side on which the driver's seatbelt lies.

87   D – Flail chest

The paradoxical chest wall movements are characteristic of flail chest, which is associated with respiratory distress.

88   A – Aortic dissection/disruption

The rapid deceleration as a mechanism of injury, coupled with the immediate decompensation and loss of radial pulses prior to arrest in this patient, are signs of aortic dissection. This is an injury that results in death at the scene, usually before the arrival of emergency services.

89   E – Haemothorax

The decreased air entry and chest wall expansion suggest a haemothorax or pneumothorax; the lack of tracheal deviation rules out tension pneumothorax, and the dull percussion is a sign of haemothorax.

90   I – Tracheobronchial injury

Both the rapid deceleration injury and the fact that the patient has stridor and subcutaneous emphysema point to a rupture of the tracheobronchial tree.

91   H – Tension pneumothorax

This man has a flail chest. The positive intrathoracic pressure produced by intubation and artificial ventilation is likely to have caused a tension pneumothorax. Intubation in this kind of scenario is usually covered by insertion of a chest drain.

92   B – Cardiac tamponade

This is a classic picture of cardiac tamponade. Blood collects in the pericardium, causing muffled heart sounds, increased CVP and decreased systolic BP. Aspiration of as little as 15 ml of blood can produce significant symptomatic relief.

93   I – Tracheobronchial tree injury

The chest drain is in the correct position. Despite this, there is evidence of a large air leak, given the increasing size of the pneumothorax. Tracheobronchial injury is likely. This may require insertion of more than one chest drain until definitive treatment can be achieved.

STERILISATION

94   E – Irradiation

This type of equipment is mass-produced and can be sterilised industrially in large batches by irradiation.

95   D – Glutaraldehyde

This type of equipment is heat-sensitive and requires rapid disinfection between patients in the clinic. Glutaraldehyde can rapidly accomplish this.

96   C – Ethylene oxide

Sutures are both single-use and heat-sensitive, and ethylene oxide can provide sterilisation without affecting the suture material.

97   B – Dry heat

The fine blades of these scissors are very sensitive to corrosion, so a method of sterilisation which does not involve moisture must be used.

TOURNIQUETS

98   B – Simple tourniquet

This procedure requires only a simple tourniquet, to isolate only the digit being operated on; isolation of the whole limb is not required.

99   D – Tourniquet at 200 mmHg

This is a procedure on the upper limb which requires a tourniquet, and in the upper limb tourniquets should be inflated to 50 mmHg over the systolic blood pressure.

100   A – No tourniquet

This is a procedure which would usually require a tourniquet, but the patient has a past history of peripheral vascular disease, which means a tourniquet cannot be used.

BIOPSY TECHNIQUES

101 F – Frozen section

This situation requires an immediate result during the operation.

102 E – Fine-needle aspiration cytology

The thyroid is easily accessible, and even though architectural data cannot be gained from this technique; if the result is follicular cells, a lobectomy can be performed.

103 D – Excisional biopsy

Excisional biopsies are usually performed for skin lesions.

104 C – Endoscopic biopsy

This type of lesion can be accessed with a cystoscope to take a sample for a biopsy.

PAROTID SWELLINGS

105   D – Pleomorphic adenoma

Pleomorphic adenomas are more common in men between 40 and 60 years of age. They are slow-growing, painless and usually unilateral.

106   C – Adenolymphoma

Adenolymphomas (Warthin's tumour) are more common in men between 60 and 80 years of age. They are painless. Approximately 10% are bilateral and these are usually asynchronous.

107   H – Squamous cell carcinoma

Squamous cell carcinomas are more common in men and those who have had prior irradiation. They are rapidly growing and aggressive. They are also painful and tend to affect the facial nerve.

108   J – Frey syndrome

Frey syndrome or gustatory sweating can occur after surgery to the parotid gland. Flushing and sweating usually occur along the distribution of the auriculotemporal nerve. Damage to this nerve has been postulated to be a cause.

109   I – Acute viral sialadenitis

Acute viral sialadenitis, better known as mumps, causes orchitis in 20% of post-pubertal men. Mumps can be distinguished from other forms of acute parotitis by the absence of a neutrophil leucocytosis.

110   G – Sjögren syndrome

Secondary Sjögren syndrome is associated with connective tissue disorders such as SLE and rheumatoid arthritis. Its features consist of dry eyes and a dry mouth.

111   K – Mikulicz syndrome

Mikulicz syndrome is a triad consisting of symmetrical enlargement of all salivary glands, narrowing of the palpebral fissures secondary to lacrimal gland enlargement and parchment-like dryness of the mouth. In Mikulicz syndrome there is enlargement of the glands secondary to leukaemia or generalised disease. It is due to an autoimmune process in the salivary glands.

112   F – Sialolithiasis

Stone formation in the salivary glands usually occurs in the submandibular gland, but can occur in any of the glands. Just before meals, salivation is stimulated, causing saliva to build up behind the obstruction, resulting in swelling and increased pain.

JOINT INFECTIONS

113   C – *Haemophilus influenzae*

Haemophilus influenzae is three times more common a cause of septic arthritis than *Staphylococcus aureus* in children aged under 5 years.

114   E – *Staphylococcus aureus*

Staphylococcus aureus is the most common cause of septic arthritis in children aged over 5 years.

115   E – *Staphylococcus aureus*

Staphylococcus aureus is the most common cause of osteomyelitis in children aged over 5 years and in adults.

SUTURE MATERIALS

116 D – 6-0 Prolene

The distal portion of a femoro-distal anastomosis requires very small sutures. In vascular surgery a smooth monofilament non-absorbable suture is used.

117 A – 1 PDS

Large, absorbable sutures are required to provide strength for a mass abdominal closure.

118 C – 3-0 Prolene

A non-absorbable monofilament suture.

119 F – Steel wire

Steel wire is required to provide strength in sternal closure.

120 B – 3-0 PDS

Absorbable monofilament used on an atraumatic round-bodied needle to perform a single-layer interrupted seromuscular anastomosis as recommended by the Royal College of Surgeons.

MULTIPLE ENDOCRINE NEOPLASIA

121 A – Gorlin syndrome

The patient has a marfanoid appearance, which is associated with MEN IIB, Gorlin syndrome.

122 B – Sipple syndrome

Type IIA MEN, Sipple syndrome, is associated with phaeochromocytoma in 20–50%, and these are commonly bilateral.

123 C – Werner syndrome

Pituitary adenoma and parathyroid hyperplasia are common in MEN type I, Werner syndrome, which has an autosomal dominant inheritance.

124 A – Gorlin syndrome

Type IIB MEN, Gorlin syndrome, is associated with multiple mucosal neuromas.

TYPES OF GRAFT

125 A – Allogenic heterotropic graft

Kidneys are transplanted to a different anatomical location in the recipient.

126 E – Xenogenic orthotopic graft

This is a transplant between two species.

127 C – Autogenic graft

This transplant is from one site on an individual to another site in the same individual.

128 A – Allogenic heterotropic graft

The pancreas is transplanted to a different anatomical location in the recipient.

Allografts are grafts from a member of a species to another of the same species. Autografts are grafts from one site on an individual to another site. Xenografts are grafts from a member of a species to a member of another species. Orthotopic grafts are transplanted to the normal anatomical site in the donor. Heterotopic grafts are transplanted to a different anatomical site.

UPPER GASTROINTESTINAL HAEMORRHAGE

129 D – Gastric ulcer

Gastric ulcer is more common in elderly patients. It is associated with pain brought on by food, and often weight loss secondary to this. It is also associated with NSAID use.

130 E – Mallory–Weiss tear

Mallory–Weiss tears are associated with retching prior to the onset of haematemesis and with alcohol excess.

131 F – Oesophageal varices

The patient has stigmata of liver disease which are associated with variceal haemorrhage, which typically causes large bleeds.

132 B – Duodenal ulcer

Duodenal ulcers are more common in young men who smoke and are associated with pain relieved by eating.

133 A – Aorto-enteric fistula

Aorto-enteric fistulae are a known late complication following AAA repair.

LOWER GASTROINTESTINAL HAEMORRHAGE

134 A – Angiodysplasia

Recurrent painless episodes of rectal bleeding or a single large bleed can be the presentation of this condition. The telangiectasia point to Osler–Weber–Rendu syndrome, which is associated with angiodysplasia.

135 G – Ulcerative colitis

The age of this patient and the presence of mucus accompanying the alteration in bowel habit and crampy pain are features of inflammatory bowel disease. Clubbing is also associated with inflammatory bowel disease. Bleeding is more common in ulcerative colitis.

136 D – Diverticular disease

Diverticular disease is common in patients over 60, and its incidence increases with age. The length of the history with no associated weight loss and the left-sided pain relieved by defecation make the diagnosis of diverticular disease more likely than that of colorectal cancer.

137 B – Colorectal cancer

This patient has lost weight over a very short period of time, coupled with an alteration in bowel habit and rectal bleeding. These are all sinister features suggesting malignancy.

138 E – Haemorrhoids

Haemorrhoids are more common in pregnancy and are associated with fresh blood on the toilet paper, and not mixed with stool.

FLUIDS

139 H – 142 mmol/l

140 G – 130 mmol/l

141 I – 154 mmol/l

142 E – 30 mmol/l

143 A – 0 mmol/l

The concentrations are shown in the table below.

Table 3

Fluid	Sodium concentration (mmol/l)	Potassium concentration (mmol/l)
Serum	142	4.5
Normal saline	154	0
Dextrose saline	30	0
5% dextrose	0	0
Hartmann's	130	5
Gelofusine	154	0

HYPOVOLAEMIC SHOCK

144 B – Class II hypovolaemic shock

145 A – Class I hypovolaemic shock

146 C – Class III hypovolaemic shock

The features of the different classes of hypovolaemic shock are shown in the table below.

Table 4

	Class I	Class II	Class III	Class IV
Pulse	< 100	> 100	> 120	> 140
Blood pressure	Normal	Normal	Decreased	Decreased
Pulse pressure	Normal	Decreased	Decreased	Decreased
Respiratory rate	14–20	20–30	30–40	> 40

NUTRITIONAL SUPPORT

147   C – Nasojejunal feeding

This condition will require medium-term feeding, and needs a method which infuses food distal to the pancreas.

148   E – PEG feeding

PEG feeding is the best option for long-term feeding.

149   A – Jejunostomy

Indications for jejunostomy include major upper abdominal surgery, major abdominal trauma, post-operative chemotherapy or radiotherapy and malnourished patients undergoing abdominal surgery.

150   F – TPN

There is no other appropriate route but TPN, as the small bowel is affected.

THYROID NEOPLASMS

151   F – Papillary carcinoma

Papillary carcinoma is characterised by psammoma bodies. It is more common in women aged 20–50 years.

152   A – Anaplastic carcinoma

Anaplastic carcinoma presents more commonly in the older patient and is aggressive, often presenting with dysphagia, dysphonia or stridor.

153   D – Medullary carcinoma

The raised calcitonin level indicates medullary carcinoma.

NIPPLE DISCHARGE

154   C – Intraductal papilloma

This is a benign neoplasm associated with bloody single-duct discharge.

155   D – Periductal mastitis

Periductal mastitis is strongly associated with smoking; it causes a purulent discharge.

156   A – Ductal carcinoma in situ

A bloody discharge should be assumed to be from a malignancy until proved otherwise.

157   F – Prolactinoma

Essential lactation unrelated to childbirth and the systemic symptoms are consistent with the cause of the discharge being part of an endocrine process.

SHOULDER PAIN

158 A – Acute calcific tendonitis

This condition arises without injury, and is acutely and very painful. It is more common in women and in those in their third or fourth decades.

159 B – Acute dislocation

The player has sustained a direct blow, causing an acute dislocation, which is characterised by flattening of the normal shape of the deltoid.

160 C – Frozen shoulder

Frozen shoulder often presents following minor trauma in elderly people. The pain is often worse at night, and abduction and external rotation are the movements worst affected.

ASA GRADING – CLASSIFICATION OF PHYSICAL STATUS

161 D – Class 4

162 B – Class 2

163 A – Class 1

164 B – Class 2

165 C – Class 3

ASA grading is used by anaesthetists to place patients in certain groups according to their pre-operative physical condition, irrespective of the type of surgery they are planned to undergo.

Class 1 – normal, healthy individual.

Class 2 – patient with mild systemic disease.

Class 3 – patient with severe systemic disease that limits activity but is not incapacitating.

Class 4 – patient with incapacitating disease that is a constant threat to life.

Class 5 – moribund patient who is not expected to survive without an operation.

STAGING OF TRANSITIONAL CELL CARCINOMA OF BLADDER

166 $H - T_{4b}$

167 $C - T_{2a}$

Staging of bladder cancer depends on how far into the bladder wall the tumour has invaded. During TURBT the tumours should be carefully resected in layers to get specimens for accurate staging and to fully remove the more superficial tumours. Staging is as follows:

T_{is} – in situ

T_a – confined to epithelium

T_1 – invading lamina propria

T_{2a} – invading superficial muscle

T_{2b} – invading deep muscle

T_{3a} – microscopic perivesical invasion

T_{3b} – macroscopic perivesical invasion

T_{4a} – invasion into adjacent organs

T_{4b} – fixed to pelvic side wall

POLYPS

168 D – Juvenile polyp

169 A – Fibroma

170 B – Hyperplastic polyp

A polyp is defined as an abnormal elevation from an epithelial surface and can be malignant or benign. Hyperplastic polyps are the most common type. They are flat and the same colour as the bowel mucosa. They do not undergo malignant change. Juvenile polyps are typically found in children under the age of 10 years. They are usually present in the rectum but can be found anywhere in the large bowel. They are also not pre-malignant. Fibromas are rare colonic tumours arising from the submucosal layer. They are hard, mobile and pedunculated and rarely undergo malignant change. Peutz-Jeghers polyps are associated with the familial disorder and are associated with buccal hyperpigmentation. The polyps are most commonly found in the small bowel and are usually multiple. They have a low-grade malignant potential.

RADIOLOGICAL APPEARANCES

171   F – Sigmoid volvulus

172   G – Ulcerative colitis

Sigmoid volvulus is identified as a loop of distended bowel and the 'beak sign' on instant enema. Features indicating ulcerative colitis are loss of haustral fold pattern, mucosal irregularity, tubular ('lead pipe') shaped colon and the absence of faecal residue within the affected segment of bowel. Intramural gas is a sign of necrotising enterocolitis, which affects neonates. Hirschsprung's disease can be diagnosed by the presence of of a 'cone' between the collapsed distal and dilated proximal bowel on contrast enema – due to the portion of aganglionic bowel. Duodenal atresia is also seen in newborns and is picked up by the presence of a 'double bubble' on abdominal X-ray, which consists of an air-filled stomach and first part of the duodenum. Diverticular disease cannot be diagnosed on plain abdominal X-ray but often appears as segmental lumen narrowing and tethered mucosa on gastrografin enema.

PERIPHERAL NERVE INJURY

173   A – Axillary nerve

The axillary nerve is damaged in up to 5% of dislocations of the shoulder, and damage to the nerve leads to sensory loss in the 'regimental patch' area. This is on the lateral aspect of the arm, around the lower border of the deltoid muscle.

174   D – Posterior interosseous nerve of the forearm

The posterior interosseous nerve passes around the neck of the radius and is susceptible to injury here. It supplies most of the extensors of the wrist and fingers, although the extensor carpi radialis longus is supplied by the radial nerve before it divides, so some wrist extension remains. The posterior interosseous nerve is purely motor, so no sensation is lost.

175   A – Axillary nerve

The axillary nerve wraps around the surgical neck of the humerus and is susceptible to injury here. It supplies the deltoid muscle, so damage to this nerve limits abduction.

176   F – Ulnar nerve

The ulnar nerve runs just behind the medial epicondyle. Damage to the nerve produces a typical 'claw' hand, with unopposed action of the extensors and paralysis of the deep flexors to the ring and little fingers in conjunction with paralysis of the lumbricals and interossei.

177   B – Median nerve

The median nerve crosses the brachial artery anteriorly in the arm. Hence pulsatile bleeding suggesting brachial artery damage is likely to damage the median nerve.

Index